INTERMITTENT FASTING FOR WOMEN

Have You Heard of The Multiple Benefits of Intermittent Fasting but Don't Know Where to Start? Learn Fasting's Best Kept Secrets & Maximize Weight Loss in Just 30 Days

Table of Contents

Introduction 5

Chapter One The History of Intermittent Fasting 7
   How Intermittent Fasting Works and Why It Is Healthy 8
   The Hidden Benefits of Intermittent Fasting 16
   Intermittent Fasting and Cancer Patients 19

Chapter Two What Is Hunger and How to Get Past the Feeling of It 23
   How to Use Healthy Snacks to Help Adjust 25
   Hanger and Hanxiety 26
   Common Myths 27
   Common Mistakes 30
   The Myth of Breakfast — Is It Really the Most Important Meal of the Day? 32
   How Intermittent Fasting Can Slow Down Aging Process 34

Chapter Three The Lean Gain Method 35
   Getting Started With Intermittent Fasting 36
   Guidelines While Breaking Your Fast 38
   The Four Main Types of Fasting 39
   Special Advice for Overweight Women and Intermittent Fasting 42
   Children and Intermittent Fasting 44
   Long-Term and Negative Effects 45

Chapter Four Evaluate Your Progress 48
   Finding Your Suitable Eating Portion 48
   Is Intermittent Fasting for You? 48
   When to Stop Intermittent Fasting 49

Pregnancy and Fasting.. *50*

Polycystic Ovarian Syndrome and Intermittent Fasting *51*

Overcoming Binging.. *51*

Adjusting Your Intermittent Fasting Schedule *52*

Chapter Five   How to Get the Best Out of Intermittent Fasting 53

Cardio — Running, Cycling, and Swimming to Help with Intermittent Fasting Results *57*

Strength Training and Intermittent Fasting *58*

Meditation and Mindfulness *59*

Combining Intermittent Fasting with Other Diets *61*

Essential Oils to Help with Intermittent Fasting and Weight Loss *66*

The Buddy System *68*

Supplements and Vitamins to Aid in Fasting *69*

Alcohol and Intermittent Fasting *72*

Pop or Soda and Intermittent Fasting *72*

Chapter Six **73**

Three Simple and Easy Recipes for Breakfast *73*

Three Simple and Easy Recipes for Lunch *76*

Three Simple and Easy Recipes for Dinner *77*

Super Foods and Intermittent Fasting *81*

Conclusion **85**

Introduction

Welcome to the world of intermittent fasting!

Intermittent fasting simply means not eating for a designated period of time or a set number of hours and then eating during a time restricted feeding period. While the act of fasting has been around thousands of years, in the last several years, more and more women are engaging in the lifestyle of intermittent fasting. Intermittent fasting is proving to be highly beneficial to women health. There are countless benefits to participating in the lifestyle. Unlike the traditional diet, it focuses more on when you eat as opposed to what you eat. There are many ways to use fasting to your benefit and various techniques.

In recent culture, intermittent fasting has become increasingly popular. There has been research to support the practice. There is evidence of benefits on many body systems including slowing down aging, better cardiac health, better focus, weight loss, and multiple other benefits. While the vast majority of women are interested in intermittent fasting for the aid in weight loss, this guide goes over the other perks of the lifestyle, as well. Unfortunately, there is some negative stigma surrounding intermittent fasting. We have been programmed to think we need to eat six meals a day and be constantly snacking. Sadly, this is based on old, outdated science. More recent science has shown quite the opposite. There are numerous recent studies that show how effective intermittent fasting can be for your overall health. There are many different types of fasting with each having their own benefits.

This guide is to help you decide which fasting protocol is best for you and to help you understand how it works, the common myths, struggles and benefits, as well as guidelines for practices that can aid you in fasting and help you to be successful if and when you choose to endeavor into the program of intermittent fasting. There is information about special circumstances and intermittent fasting such as pregnancy, PCOS, diabetes, and for weight loss as well as tools and tricks to help you get through your hunger and onto the roads of a healthier lifestyle!

Chapter One

The History of Intermittent Fasting

Fasting has been around nearly as long as mankind itself. There are many old written sources that have shown that "starvation" has been used in various cultures, countries, and ancient civilizations to help the body recover and restore itself. It seems they were taking advantage of the benefits long before modern times. Ancient India, Greece, and Rome, in particular, used intermittent fasting, not only to strengthen the body but also to help prevent diseases. Back in ancient times, when hunting and berry gathering was one of the main sources of food, there were periods of time where nothing could be found, so natural fasting took place. Involuntary fasting caused the hunters and gatherers to be inadvertently and greatly strengthened by the gaps in sustenance. The ancient Greeks particularly believed medical treatments and cures could be found and were observed in nature. When humans, dogs, cats, and most animals are sick, they do not want to eat. This is considered the internal physician in some cultures; it is believed that the body is instinctually fasting to help to heal its self. The ancient Greeks also believed fasting helped to improve mental and cognitive function. This makes sense if you think about when you eat a big meal and feel sleepy and tired or have "food coma" as many like to call it, versus when you are fasting and your brain hyper-focuses on the task at hand. The practices of controlled starvation are key in many of the world's religions, proving self-control, and penitence. Many religions practice fasting for periods such as Ramadan in the Islamic culture where they do not eat from sunup to sundown. Christianity recognizes the forty days of lent, which represents the time that Jesus Christ fasted. Fasting is recognized in Islamic religions, Buddhism, Christianity, and countless others.

Ramadan is an Islamic tradition that is practiced by Muslims. During Ramadan, they fast during the daylight hours, finally eating only once the sun has set. While it sounds terrible at first, many reports they actually feel better after a few days of the practice. This is because they adjust to the schedule and their bodies learn to adapt to no food for a time period. This is exactly what intermittent fasting is about.

However, in more recent years, there has been scientific research discovering and confirming the various benefits of intermittent fasting for women. Science is now beginning to prove what was already known in ancient times. The multiple and seemingly endless benefits keep climbing. The benefits include slowing down the aging process, sharper focus, weight loss, better cardiac health, there is evidence it both reduces the chances of cancer and helps your body to fight it off and a wide range of other advantages, with little consequences to the practice.

Studies on Mice and Rats

There have been a growing number of studies done on mice and rats that show rather promising results with intermittent fasting. They have shown evidence of decreased aging with better stem cell rejuvenation. The studies have shown good results with fighting certain cancers by helping to better target the immune response and there have been various other studies involving weight loss and diabetic patients. Generally, mice and rats have very similar anatomy and organ systems as humans. Since our systems are so similar to mice and rats, the good results in the lab animals is a very good sign that there will be positive results in humans as well.

How Intermittent Fasting Works and Why It Is Healthy

All intermittent fasting means, in the simplest terms, is that you go through an extended period without eating. It can range from a few hours to several days. Most people stick to fasts that last somewhere between twelve and twenty hours. The time you are not eating or fasting is known as your fasting window. The time that you are not fasting is called your feeding period.

The fasting window is only for drinking water, black coffee, herbal teas, and sparkling water; any beverages with sugar, fat, or additives will break the fast. Especially starting out, it is important to maintain a fast for the time period that was set. When you consume food or eat a meal, your body spends several hours processing the meal you just ate, burning what it can from the food you consumed. Because you just ate food, it is easy to burn, and an available energy for it to break down. Your body will break down the food you just consumed instead of the fat you already have stored. This is especially true if you have just eaten food with a lot of sugar and carbohydrates. Sugars and carbs are easy to break down and convert into energy.

While you are on a fast, your body is more likely to break down and convert to energy the fat your body already has stored, as you are no longer giving it simple easy fuel. When you are in a fast, your body naturally lowers its blood sugar and insulin levels. The lower your insulin is, the less you will feel hungry and the less you will crave food. There are other reasons why intermittent fasting is considered healthy. It naturally strengthens the body and helps it to fight diseases more efficiently. Intermittent fasting also has many effects on the body systems, glands, and hormones. Most of them being positive effects. There has been evidence of fasting helping diabetics naturally regulate their insulin as well as many positive metabolic effects. To put it in the simplest terms, intermittent fasting works so well because it encourages the body into a state of ketosis, where it is burning the fat that it already has stored instead of newly consumed foods for energy. This is also what makes intermittent fasting healthy and beneficial. The best part is it is a lifestyle more than it is a diet, as it does not restrict what you eat, just the time period that you are eating.

The Hormones, Systems, and Organs Involved and Affected in Intermittent Fasting

To understand how intermittent fasting works, it is important to understand the major hormones and body systems that are affected by it. Several of the metabolic hormones are involved in a period of fasting as well as when you end a fast. These hormones include insulin, leptin, ghrelin, the human growth hormone, and several other hormones, organs, glands, and systems. Each hormone has a different purpose and they all come together to create the metabolism. Most women prefer a fast metabolism as that promotes a lower weight. Intermittent fasting is known for helping the metabolism and hormones self-regulate for a healthier body overall.

- The metabolism and intermittent fasting.

The metabolism is essentially a word used to describe the series of chemical reactions involved in sustaining life, in any and all organisms. There are three major purposes of the metabolism. These purposes are converting food into fuel so that cellular processes can adequately run, converting fuel and food into building blocks for proteins, lipids, and nucleic acids, and the elimination of nitrogenous wastes. The metabolism is basically the sum of all the chemical reaction that occurs in the body and include digestion and transporting substances from one cell to another.

A common misconception with intermittent fasting is that it significantly slows down the metabolism. Shockingly enough, however, there is some more recent research that suggests that intermittent fasting has the same or less negative effects on the metabolism when compared to regular, traditional dieting. The reasoning behind the belief that intermittent fasting helps to improve the metabolism is that there is less lean body mass loss, and the body enters the phase of fat burning. While it is not possible to lose weight without losing some amount of lean body mass, fewer seemed to be lost with intermittent fasting as opposed to traditional calorie and carb restricting diets. To preserve more of the body's lean body mass, the calorie burning of the body slows down some. Short fasting periods, however, encourage the body to tap into its own fat stores and burn a larger amount of fat stores and mass for energy. Basically, it seems that there are two major factors that make intermittent fasting compatible with most metabolisms. One being that the fasting is indeed intermittent, meaning no more than a day and that you are still providing the body with adequate nutrition in the feeding windows.

- Insulin — the 'feed me' hormone.

Our body systems react to consuming food (energy consumption) by producing insulin. Insulin is a hormone produced by the pancreas that regulates the amount of glucose in the blood. The more you eat, especially carbs and sugar, the more insulin your body produces and the less your body converts its own fats to energy. It is important for your body to be sensitive to insulin as the more sensitive your body is to the hormone, the more efficiently you will be able to use the food you consume. Insulin is also the hormone that tells you are hungry. So frequently people are feeding the cycle of eating, and then the insulin tells your body that it is hungry when really it does not need food at that time. Staying sensitive to insulin is vital maintaining a good rhythm in your fasting protocol. Once you have adjusted to intermittent fasting, your body's insulin will naturally be lowered and will stabilize. Once your insulin stabilizes, you will feel hungry much less often. Many women have stated that the first several days were difficult but after that, they simply stopped feeling hungry. All these effects are because of the natural regulation of the body's insulin. Keeping insulin lowered naturally is also proving to be extremely beneficial to type two diabetic patients. They are able to control their insulin much better simply by adjusting when they eat.

- Leptin — the 'stop eating' hormone.

Leptin is another hormone affected in intermittent fasting. Leptin is the hormone that tells you when to stop eating. Low leptin leads to an increase in hunger, which can lead to easily overeating. Generally, slender or lean individuals have low levels of leptin while heavy or obese individuals have high levels of leptin. The trouble with having high levels of leptin chronically is that leptin resistance develops. Much like insulin resistance develops when someone has chronically high insulin. When evaluated long-term, leptin is regulated by the total amount of fat mass in the body. A sharp drop in leptin can also have a poor effect on other hormones, and the rate of your metabolism in general. Intermittent fasting helps to regulate and encourage healthy levels of leptin, so it will become easier to maintain a healthy metabolism.

- Blood Glucose

Blood glucose is also known as blood sugar and is a hormone that is a simple sugar. Blood glucose is stored in the liver and skeletal system and is considered a primary energy source in the human species. Blood glucose is vital to the proper function of various organs, most importantly the brain. The brain alone can consume up to sixty percent of glucose in a fasted individual. The human body cannot use blood glucose as energy, so when enough insulin is not produced, the body converts its already stored fat into energy. A ketogenic diet is based on hypoglycemia or when your body is running on low blood sugar. This keeps the body constantly burning fat which results in the often-desired weight loss and lower fat mass in the body.

- Ghrelin — the 'you fed me at this time yesterday' hormone.

Ghrelin is a tricky little hormone that is responsible for telling your body to eat at the same time every day. With intermittent fasting, your ghrelin levels have to adjust and stabilize, which can often take a few days. Ghrelin is also sometimes responsible for making people irritable or 'hangry' while they are adjusting to the altered hormone levels. The best thing to remind yourself when struggling to regulate is that it will pass.

- The Human Growth Hormone

The human growth hormone (HGH) is increased when intermittent fasting protocols are engaged in the body. It has been proven that they can increase as much as five times the average. When the human growth hormone is increased, it produces more blood glucose, which helps to control hunger more easily. The human growth hormone helps with many body functions and the excess that intermittent fasting causes are beneficial in many ways. The human growth hormone can also actually speed up body repair as well. Because the human growth hormones drive muscle synthesis, it helps to speed up the healing process and allows you to recover from workouts and injuries quicker.

- Female hormonal effects.

There is some controversy surrounding the effects of intermittent fasting on the female hormones. One potential consequence is that intermittent fasting can "turn off" the ovaries and the reproductive hormones. When you look at the human female body objectively, it is designed for reproduction. When you practice intermittent fasting and reach a fat burning state, it sometimes causes the reproductive system to shut off temporarily. The body realizes that it is using up the fat reserves and tells the reproductive system that it is not being fed correctly and that it is therefore not suitable for childbirth. This can stop a woman's menstrual cycle. Even though you know in your mind that you will eat again, on a cellular and hormonal level, your body does not know that, so it engages in this survival mode. This does not happen to all women and if you begin missing your periods, you should consider adjusting your fasting and feeding cycles. It is always wise to discuss with a physician as well. Early onset menopause caused by this phenomenon is not something that should be taken lightly. Early onset menopause is one of the few occurrences that can happen that may mean the intermittent fasting lifestyle is not compatible with your body and reproductive system.

- The thyroid and intermittent fasting.

Intermittent fasting can have both positive and negative effects on the thyroid. The thyroid is a gland, located in the neck, that is responsible for secreting hormones that regulate the growth rate and metabolism in humans.

Women with hypothyroidism or low thyroid originally were warned to stay away from intermittent fasting and food depravation lifestyles. Recent research has shown this to be false, however. In the recent studies, it has shown that even on long-term fast, like for seven to ten days, there are not any real negative effects. However, many doctors and scientist do believe that what really affects hypo thyroids is the calorie intake. With too low of calories, the thyroid begins to struggle which means that intermittent fasting is okay for hypothyroidism because it is not actually restricting the calorie intake, just changing the intake times. While fasting can be a stress on our body, especially before it has fully adjusted to intermittent fasting, there is no recent research supporting that it is bad for those women with thyroid issues. The thyroid is a fairly sensitive gland and can cause many symptoms when it is not functioning properly. Often, the root causes of thyroid issues could be autoimmune, lack of proper nutrients that help the thyroid, increased stress hormones and cortisol can also exasperate the thyroid functions, the infection can affect the thyroids as well as poor digestion. Low stomach acid and low enzymes can affect it as well. Essentially, if you have a thyroid issue and want to engage in intermittent fasting, it is generally okay if you follow the simple guidelines. These include getting enough nutrition and calories and making sure your digestive system is adequate.

For a healthy thyroid, fasting does not negatively affect the thyroid. Thyroid hormones, one of them being T3. T3 is the active form of thyroid. It is actually one of the hormones responsible for regulating certain functions of your body. T3 is responsible for your heart rate, some components of your metabolism, and your body temperature. T4 is a prohormone. T4 is the main hormone secreted by the thyroid. T4 is important because it actually encourages the production of the T3 hormone. Then there is also TSH, or the thyroid stimulating hormone, that encourages the production of both T3 and T4. When the thyroid stimulating hormone is high, it means the body is having a hard time producing T3. After a study that was a ten-day fast, there was evidence of a slight change in the T3 hormone, however, there was none what so ever in the T4 hormone and no change in the TSH or thyroid stimulating hormone. What this meant, in the end, is that a long ten day fast messed with the active thyroid hormone a little bit, but the long-term effect was unchanged. So, all it really did was temporarily slow down the metabolism in the state of a fast. The multi-day fast changed the active thyroid but did not ultimately damage or change the ability to make T4 or TSH. What this means is that all it did was slow down the metabolism but only while they were actually fasting. Not during the time of feeding. Once the fast is broken, it actually wakes up the metabolism so fast that it compensates for slowing down during the period of fasting. Therefore, in the end, the study showed the compensation increased the metabolism. The bottom line is, while the thyroid hormones are affected during intermittent fasting, it is not necessarily negative or harmful and can actually help to speed up the metabolism.

The Hidden Benefits of Intermittent Fasting

While most people like the idea of intermittent fasting for weight loss purposes, there are numerous benefits that are not as well-known and talked about as well. To name just a few, there is the natural regulation of insulin and blood sugar (glucose); intermittent fasting helps to reduce risks of common diseases like heart disease, obesity, and diabetes; intermittent fasting helps to actually slow the body's aging; and it has been known to drastically improve focus and energy. This is especially true while on a fast. Many women have stated that their focus has never been better than it has been while mid fast.

- Benefit One: Intermittent fasting helps to naturally regulate the body's insulin and blood sugar levels.

This concept has recently had a fair amount of attention because of the great results in diabetic patients. They are able to naturally regulate their insulin levels while using intermittent fasting. This has shown to work as well, if not better than just controlling the diet and exercise. Many type two diabetics were able to use intermittent fasting solely as their means of controlling the condition.

- Benefit Two: Helps to reduce risks of very common diseases such as obesity, heart disease, and diabetes and helping to strengthen the body.

Intermittent fasting forces the body into ketosis which is also a state of fat burning. Since the body is burning fat, it is decreasing the risk factors for common diseases. Being in a fat burning state helps to release certain chemicals into the bloodstream that help to break up the bad cholesterol. The insulin is naturally lowered and regulated for diabetics and weight loss is promoted and generally achieved by the forced state of fat burning. Helping reduce illness and diseases is an age-old claim to fasting. In recent years, there seems to be quite a bit of information backing up that claim. In ancient times before obesity was a common issue and fasting was a way of life, there were significantly less heart disease and weight-related problems. A big part of this was because they lived solely on plant and meat based foods and there was natural fasting when food was not available. In recent times, however, it can be attributed as a benefit of fasting.

- Benefit Three: Helps with slowing down the aging process.

Another age-old claim to intermittent fasting is that it significantly slows down the process of aging. The science behind this claim is that fasting lowers the hormone IGF-1. This is the growth hormone that is often attributed too aging, tumor growth, and cancer risk. As people age, their intestinal stem cells begin to lose the ability to regenerate. These particular stem cells are the sources for all new intestinal cells. The age-related loss of stem cell function can simply be reversed with a twenty-four hour fast. On a recent study on mice, the researchers found that fasting dramatically increased the stem cells ability to impressively regenerate on both old and young mice. Mice and humans are quite similar anatomically so results are often the same. The cells begin breaking down fatty acids instead of glucose; this is a change that allows stem cells to become more regenerative. The slowing down of aging by allowing the stem cells to regenerate in mice has been so successful researchers are trying to come up with a medication that mimics the effects of fasting. The studies showed that not only did the stem cell regeneration slow down the aging process, it actually reversed it on a cellular level and significantly increased life longevity in the mice.

- Benefit Four: Sharper focus.

When your body is in a period of fasting, your body has to hyper-focus on the task at hand. This phenomenon occurs in a period of "starvation". It increases attention to detail and sharpens the mind. It makes sense when you think about when you eat a big meal. You generally feel sleepy and full afterward. This is where the term "food coma" comes from. You eat a big meal and want to take a nap. Intermittent fasting has the opposite effect. In a fast, your insulin is naturally low thereby giving you the ability to focus better on your task at hand. This is also the same reason that women on a ketogenic diet plan report that they have better focus and a clearer mind. The body is forced into a state of ketosis or fat burning, causing the brain to only focus on one thing at a time.

- Benefit five: Better cardiac health.

Better heart health is certainly a perk of engaging in the intermittent fasting lifestyle. The way it helps with cardiac health is that it lowers the risk factors for heart disease. Intermittent fasting aids in weight loss which helps to lower insulin and naturally regulate the body's other hormones. It can help to lower the blood pressure which can decrease the risk factors of heart attack and stroke. Intermittent fasting forces the body to burn its own fat stores which means less fat stored in the body which aids in lowered cholesterol and triglycerides. Fasting induces ketosis which helps to break down the fat stores and releases cholesterol destroying agents into the bloodstream. Better cardiac health was found in people that fasted just two days a week.

Intermittent Fasting and Cancer Patients

Intermittent fasting in cancer patients seems to have a promising future. There have been several studies done both on mice and on humans with good results. It seems that one benefit that intermittent fasting has on women is that it is helping to trigger the immune system. The immune system in humans is designed to destroy and hunt down harmful pathogens in the body. When it comes to cancer though, the body seems to be not so good at finding and killing its own altered and abnormal cells, such as cancer cells. Many of the newer cancer treatments work on targeting the development and stimulation of the body's own immune system.

Now, recent research is finding that something as simple as a fasting lifestyle could be doing the work they have been trying to develop. There was a fairly new study at a university in California that was done on lab mice. This study mostly was surrounded around mesothelioma. This experiment used lab mice that had received chemotherapy along with a fasting diet and it showed that the immune system had a significantly easier time targeting and killing off breast cancer cells and skin cancer cells. The mice produced more cells that helped the immune system when on a fasting program; these cells included B cells and T cells. These cells actively target and destroy tumor cells. Along with that discovery, they learned that the cells that often protect tumors from chemotherapy which are called T regulatory cells were not found in the tumors following this protocol, which means that the chemotherapy drugs were able to do their job much better and with fewer barriers.

The same people that did this research on mice also did a piloted study with human cancer patients. This was mostly to learn if fasting programs with chemotherapy would be safe. The use of two-day fasts, four-day fasts, and water only fasts, along with calorie-restricted diets were all found to be safe and useful to cancer patients while being supervised by physicians. All the studies also showed that a fasting or intermittent fasting diet went along well with chemotherapy and could be useful in slowing the growth of tumors in cancer patients.

The side effects in cancer patients from chemotherapy were also affected in the studies. Side effects to chemotherapy can range from minor to crippling. Intermittent fasting can help to protect the body against side effects. One of the studies showed that a patient fasted for several days before the treatment and then ate normally right before their treatment. They did not appear to lose a dangerous amount of weight and it did not have any noticeable interference with their treatments. What did come out of it was significantly reduced side effects in the patients that were active in a fasting diet program. Patients that were part of the trial had less weakness and fatigue, less nausea, fewer headaches, and no vomiting at all. They also saw a reduced amount of dry mouth, cramps, mouth sores, and numbness.

The skeptics of the intermittent fasting lifestyle are concerned that it promotes eating patterns that are not healthy and could promote eating disorders. The research behind intermittent fasting in cancer patients does not support this, however. There have been several studies that show when guided by professionals, that it is safe for cancer fighters. There is minimal evidence that long-term calorie restriction could have the potential to have some negative effects, but most of these are not significant. For women who are battling cancer, it may be worth trying. The results appear to be safe and stable there seems to be a lot of hope with it for cancer patients. Be sure to only engage in intermittent fasting though, with the approval of your doctors and oncology teams.

Fasting and the Brain: The Effects It Has and Potentially Slowing Down Neurologic Diseases

Intermittent fasting is unsurprisingly good for the brain. There is a multitude of neurochemical changes that occur in the brain during a state of fasting. Neurotrophic factors are improved along with better cognitive function, resistance to stress, and reduction of inflammation. Intermittent fasting provides your brain with a challenge and the brain adapts to the test by creating and adapting pathways of stress response that allow your brain to better deal with disease and stress risks. The changes that happen during a period of fast mimic the chemical changes in the brain that happen with regular exercise. Both exercise and periods of fasting increase and better produce protein levels in the brain which helps to promote the growth of new and healthy neurons, and helps to improve the connection between the neurons and make the synapses stronger. Fasting can help to encourage and better produce new nerve cells that come from stem cells in the hippocampus. Fasting also helps to increase and stimulate the production of ketones by the liver, which neurons in the brain use as an energy source. Fasting helps to multiply the number of mitochondria in nerve cells as well since neurons are constantly adapting to stress by producing more mitochondria. Since mitochondria in the neurons are increased, the ability for new neurons to form and keep the connections between the neurons also is improved which ultimately leads to improving the abilities of memory and learning capabilities. Besides the impressive capabilities of intermittent fasting improving brain function, there is also evidence that intermittent has the ability to help enhance nerve cells to aid in the repair of DNA. The results of several studies showed that intermittent fasting helped to shift stem cells from a dormant state to self-renewal; because of this, it triggered the regeneration of organ systems based on stem cells. In conclusion, because of the mild stress fasting puts on the brain, it can help to slow down the growth of abnormal brain cells. By slowing those cells, it could potentially be slowing down or reversing the growth of cells that cause Alzheimer's and Parkinson's disease. The brain is an incredibly complex organ and it is a major breakthrough to show that something as simple as not eating for a few extra hours a day can possibly change and prevent devastating neurological diseases.

Chapter Two

What Is Hunger and How to Get Past the Feeling of It

Hunger is basically your body telling you it wants food and that you should feed it, or the desire or urge to eat. A big hurdle in intermittent fasting is overcoming the initial hunger that you feel. Basically, your mind is trying to convince you that you will die if you do not immediately eat. So it is important to convince your mind otherwise and break the cycle of immediately eating when you think you are hungry. The human body has evolved for thousands of years and is well equipped to handle significant periods of fasting. Training the mind, however, is the greater challenge. First, it is important to recognize that there are two main kinds of hunger. There is physical hunger, where your body is actually hungry and asking for food and there is psychological hunger, where your emotions are telling you they want food. It is essential to your success to be able to recognize the difference and the symptoms of physical versus psychological hunger.

Signs of physical hunger include hunger that comes on gradually and does not need to be satisfied immediately, it can be satisfied with any food, it causes satisfaction and no guilty emotions.

The signs of psychological hunger include sudden and urgent need to eat, often comes with specific cravings, leaves you feeling full to the point of discomfort, displeased with yourself, and guilt.

Getting through the hunger especially the phycological hunger in the middle of a fast can be a challenging mental obstacle. There are many good ways to try and help yourself get through the hunger. One of them is to be sure you are not mistaking hunger with dehydration.

Often, you think you are feeling pains of hunger when really your body simply wants water. Coffee and tea are excellent for helping to curb the feelings of hunger as well; sugar-free drinks are good options as well. Brushing your teeth has been proven to help reduce the hungry feelings as well. One of the best ways is to stay focused on something else and remain active. Doing something you enjoy or an activity where you are productive are easily the best hunger deterrents. It is easy for your time to fly right on by when you are engrossed in an activity and often before you know it, your fasting time has passed, anything to keep your mind engaged enough to break the craving or feelings of hunger.

Studies have shown that once your body adapts to fasting, the hormone ghrelin, which is the hormone that tells your body you what time you normally eat at, begins to adjust. Many women think that the longer you do not eat, or fast, the hungrier you become. This is false. Hunger comes and goes in a fast. After several days, your hormones begin to adjust. Many women say that the first four days are the most difficult with managing and adjusting to hunger. After about the fourth day, however, your hormones have significantly adjusted, and many have reported they become less and less hungry. Sometimes, when you are feeling hungry, it may actually be the ghrelin hormone telling you that you need salt. Sodium intake is quite important to the body. It has many critical functions in the human body. Salt is needed to help the heart function and pump adequately and is also key in cell-to-cell communication and is vital to helping the major organs function properly.

Getting through your first fast takes willpower and determination, but it does get easier. We are trained from an early age to be eating almost all the time to be healthy and lose weight. By engaging in intermittent fasting, you are retraining and conditioning your body to do something that it has forgotten it is meant to do. Fighting hunger is often the toughest battle for women who choose to endeavor on the tricky, yet beneficial route of intermittent fasting. There are also tools and techniques to help you overcome your hunger. Practicing meditation and yoga have shown to be significantly helpful in managing your feelings of hunger and recalibrating and clearing the mind. Essential oils have been shown to have positive effects on managing hunger and cravings as well. There are many tools available to help get a grip on controlling your hunger and feelings. Be sure to utilize some of them to help yourself get over this first hurdle.

How to Use Healthy Snacks to Help Adjust

Using healthy snacks is a good way to adjust to intermittent fasting. Gradually cutting out junk food and replacing them with foods that are healthy are an excellent way to prepare your body. If you are having trouble adjusting to a fasting period or are overeating when breaking a fast, using a healthy snack can really help. Make the last thing you eat before a fast be something high in good fat and low in carbs. Then make the first thing you eat after a fast be the same. You may need to gradually lengthen your fasts over time if you are just having too much trouble at first. Start with an eight hour fast and go from there. Reward yourself with a healthy snack after it. Healthy snacks are foods that are high in the good fats that will actually satisfy your hunger, not just mask it. Having a nutrient dense snack is what will satisfy the feeling best.

Examples of healthy snacks:

- Avocado
- Peanuts
- Soy nuts
- A spoonful of peanut butter
- Pumpkin or sunflower seeds

Hanger and Hanxiety

The hanger is real! Originally this term was meant as a joke to describe the progressive irritation of a hungry girl, it has now become an actual term used regularly. Hanger is a common term used to describe the irritable feeling that comes with being hungry. Many people that already deal with hanger issues may really struggle the first couple of days of fasting. As with most things, it will be easier to handle if you anticipate it and are prepared to handle it. If you know you get irritable while hungry, perhaps plan to do something that you find enjoyable to distract you. Take a walk, practice mindfulness, many have found meditation to be useful when going through a rough patch in the fasting. Keep in mind that it will pass. Your body will adjust after the first three days and it does get easier. Many women have said that the best way to combat their "hanger" is with laughter. Finding a funny picture, video, book or person significantly helped the feelings to pass! Also having herbal tea, coffee, or water can help with getting passed the irritability. The feelings of hanger are not pleasant to anyone so be sure you are ready with a potential distraction should the feeling occur.

The other hunger-induced feeling that can occur is anxiety or commonly referred to as 'hanxiety'. This is the uneasy or panicked feeling you have induced by hunger. It is essentially stress-induced anxiety. As with the angry, agitated feelings, it will pass. If you are prone to anxiety, be prepared with activities that you know will distract and relax you. Hunger induced anxiety is unpleasant and can be alarming. While not quite as common as a hanger, hunger-induced anxiety is a real feeling and should be treated appropriately. Many women have found that yoga, Pilates, or exercise can significantly help their anxiety as well as the earlier mentioned meditation, mindfulness exercises, headspace, essential oils and various other anxiety coping tools are helpful with getting through it. Just always remember that it is not permanent and you will adjust. If anxiety is a preexisting condition for you, it may be a good idea to consult with your doctor first and discuss ways to help you cope with the adjustment to minimize your anxiety and cause the least amount of stress on your mind and body systems.

Common Myths

As with any dieting or lifestyle change, there are always common myths and misconceptions that seem to accompany them. Debunking the common myths is important to better the understanding of the intermittent fasting concepts. When you first begin telling people what you are doing, in all likely hood someone will say that they have heard something bad about it. Since you have done your research, you know that the majority of the negative claims are in fact, false and that intermittent fasting is highly beneficial in a wide variety of ways. The most common myths are as follows: fasting is unnatural and unhealthy; it slows the metabolic rate; it causes loss of muscle tone; it can cause eating disorders and encourages overeating; and that you cannot exercise while fasting.

Myth One - Fasting Is Unnatural and Unhealthy for the Human Body

How false this myth is! Fasting is extremely natural. As stated before, in ancient and even stone age times, there were natural periods of fasting when meat could not be hunted, and berries and plants could not be gathered. This meant that people simply did not eat. Not only is intermittent fasting quite natural, but it is also even considered healthy. Humans are quite well adapted to long fasts because of the reasons above. This myth can certainly be debunked simply by history. Besides intermittent fasting being historically inaccurate, there are now studies and testimonies of the benefits of the intermittent fasting lifestyle.

Myth Two - Intermittent Fasting Slows Down the Metabolism

Intermittent fasting slowing down the metabolism is also an inaccurate claim. Intermittent fasting actually speeds up the metabolism because it naturally lowers the insulin and blood sugar. So really, intermittent fasting helps to regulate the hormones that affect your metabolism which is part of why it is so successful with weight loss.

Myth Three - Intermittent Fasting Causes Muscle Loss

Unless done incorrectly on a very thin person, intermittent fasting causing any significant muscle loss is unlikely. The event in which this could take place is if the body has no fat stores left and begins to eat muscle. This is highly unlikely though. Intermittent fasting does not cause serious muscle loss or breakdown when used correctly. There is some controversy that doing too much cardio while fasting can cause some minor breakdown of muscle tissues, but there are little science and research to back these claims. While anytime there is weight loss, there is generally some mild degree of muscle loss, though it is easily built back up with proper supplements and exercise.

Myth Four - Intermittent Fasting Causes Eating Disorders

If you have already struggled with anorexia or bulimia, fasting may not be for you. While it certainly does not cause eating disorders, you do not want to fall in too poor diet habits on accident. If you have a history of an eating disorder, talk to your doctor or therapist about the healthiest way to proceed with the intermittent fasting program. Planning and cooking meals and snacks ahead of time may be quite helpful with this, same with having a meal and eating plan that you stick too is helpful. Having a strong support system is especially important if you have previously overcome an eating disorder. Though as stated above, intermittent fasting does not cause eating disorders.

Myth Five - Intermittent Fasting Encourages Overeating

If you break your fast correctly and stick to simple rules, overeating should not typically occur. Intermittent fasting actually shrinks down the stomach which theoretically leaves the body craving less food. Especially if you break your fast with a food high in good fat, then it breaks down fat first which leaves you feeling more satisfied. The majority of all overeating is typically psychological. The other reason that this is false is that because intermittent fasting naturally lowers the blood sugar and insulin levels, it leaves you feeling less hungry because of the stability in the blood sugars. While the first few days can be rough, ultimately you should crave much less food. While your body is in the adjustment period, this is generally when the most overeating occurs. Typically, after adjusting to a more constricted stomach, people often feel uncomfortably full once they begin eating after a fast and do not want to have large meals or eat too much.

Myth Six - You Cannot Exercise While in a Fast

Not being able to exercise while in a fast is another common misconception. Many people fast all night and through midday if they are on a sixteen-hour fast, eight-hour feeding schedule. A fair amount of research states that doing your exercise first thing in the morning is the ideal time to work out, and this technically puts you in the middle of your fast. Many women actually work out in replace of breakfast. They have reported that working out first thing in the morning helps them wake up and prepare them for the day far more adequately than their previous morning habits. Since fasting does not necessarily alter your diet, just when you eat, your workout habits should not need to be drastically adjusted. The only time when you may want to go easy on working out is when you are first adjusting either to intermittent fasting itself or adjusting to a ketogenic diet. In these cases, it is recommended to rest and allow the adjustment period, as to help with avoiding keto flu symptoms and overstressing of the body systems.

Once you are appropriately adjusted, however, exercise will aid in weight loss and an overall healthier diet. The one string of truth to this myth is that it may be unwise to do exceptionally intense workouts while in a fast. There are chances you may get some muscle breakdown if the intensity is too high for a fasted work out.

Common Mistakes

With every diet or lifestyle change, there are common mistakes that can alter your potential success. Intermittent fasting is not a clear or precise art; there are many variables that can affect your results. There are, however, simple mistakes that can damage your results that are quite easily preventable. Many do not even realize they are making them. Being aware of your habits is very important to success with intermittent fasting. Like with any lifestyle change, adjustment takes time, and nobody gets it right all at once.

Not Eating Enough in the Feeding Period

Not getting enough to eat after a fast is a common mistake. The stomach has a certain amount of dispensability. Meaning it can shrink and expand to a certain amount. While in a fast, it contracts and adapts to handling less. When you are eating a lot, it expands and gets used to accommodate larger amounts of food. When you are preparing to break your fast, you naturally want to eat heavy foods that are very dense. This is a common mistake because, with your stomach in a shrunken state, you quickly do not have room for the good things like vegetables and fibers. It is important to get enough foods with good fats, especially at the beginning of breaking your fast. Breaking your fast with good fats such as avocado, eggs, peanut butter is a good way to kick start your appetite and to transition the body from a self-fat burning state to burning the fats that you feed it. Maintaining enough calories is important too. When you do not get enough calories, the effects are more undesirable and detrimental. Meal planning and research can really help with this as well as planning when the best time of day to break your fast is.

Coffee and Tea Creamers

This is another common mistake that people unintentionally do that causes a break in fast without realizing it. Even a half-tablespoon of coffee creamer or almond milk is enough to trigger an insulin response and break a fast. As soon as you include the substance in your beverage, you may as well end the fast because you will need to start over. Adjusting to coffee in black can be difficult if it is not what you are accustomed to. Many people that cannot seem to get used to it simply switch to herbal teas.

Not Drinking Enough Water

Another common mistake is simply not keeping yourself hydrated enough. Many times, when you feel like you may be hungry, it may actually be your body telling you to hydrate it. Women were shocked to find that many hunger pains during a fast were curbed by simply drinking water or tea. The body also demands more salt on an intermittent fasting diet. Be sure to get enough water and salt as these are essential to getting good, healthy results. Drinking enough water and staying well hydrated also helps to prevent and get over the keto flu, if you are also following the ketogenic diet. Hydration is key to any change in diet and will nearly always improve your results.

Not Having Enough Support

Often times with any diet this is the biggest cause of failure. Support for a life change is absolutely a necessity. Without having a support system to lean on, ask questions and discuss ideas with, most people are not successful. If you are struggling and frustrated, be sure to find someone who is also going through the changes and adjustments that come with changing your habits to an intermittent fasting lifestyle.

There are many online support groups with great support systems and knowledge to share. Changing your life is hard as it is and it is nearly impossible to do alone.

The Myth of Breakfast — Is It Really the Most Important Meal of the Day?

From a young age, it has been drilled into our heads that breakfast is the most important meal of the day; however, the more research that comes out regarding intermittent fasting is beginning to tell us that breakfast may not be as beneficial and necessary as we are programmed to think. Over time, it has been proven that there is no real negative effect or significance to skipping breakfast. The pesky little hormone of ghrelin is partially responsible for putting us in the habit of eating breakfast every morning. This is the hormone that tells us to eat at the same time every day. Part of why we feel we need to eat breakfast is that it is simply a habit ingrained in our brains and in our hormones for most of our lives.

Individuals have recently found that once they adapted and retrained their bodies to not be expecting to be fed first thing in the morning, that there were actually little to no negative effects in their daily lives and routines. To put it in simple terms, our bodies naturally fast overnight, eating breakfast is breaking the fast first thing in the morning and it is not necessarily at a benefit. Individuals who skipped breakfast were also shown to have burned more calories during the day as opposed to those that ate breakfast in the morning. In the morning, as we have theoretically fasted overnight unless you are a sleepwalking eater, you are already in or near a mild state of ketosis, as your blood glucose stores have been depleted overnight. Within several hours of waking up, our body hormones will adopt that will make it stronger in the long run. The growth hormone gets released and this will help improve insulin sensitivity.

Insulin sensitivity is important to maintaining a fast comfortably and is the hormone responsible for telling you that your body wants to be fed. Staying as sensitive as possible to insulin helps to keep the blood glucose levels stable which helps you to feel less hungry and avoid overeating. If you decide skipping breakfast is not an option and you are unwilling to give it a try, it will be necessary to arrange your fasting around breakfast. However, the worst type of breakfast you can have is a high carbohydrate, sugary breakfast after breaking a fast. This throws the hormones out of balance by raising your blood glucose and causing the insulin response. It will not only completely end ketosis but will make it very difficult to reestablish it for several days. So, the bottom line is if you do not think you can skip breakfast, at the very least avoid an unhealthy one.

Many people want breakfast simply out of a lifetime of habit and breaking that routine is quite difficult at first. Many women find that working out first thing in the morning is a great way to get past the breakfast cravings. Working out in the morning is a great time to get in some exercise and wake you up for the day

Our Bodies Already Feed Us in the Morning

Ultimately, our bodies already are feeding us in the morning because you should be in a fat burning state. Once you are in a state of fat burning, it is unnecessary to eat breakfast because your body is already burning its reserved fat cell. When you wake up in the morning, you are already in a state of mild ketosis, or in the fat burning state. Eating breakfast breaks the ketosis and you go back to converting carbs for energy. Most women reported that once they adjusted to not eating breakfast in the morning, they hardly noticed a difference. The beauty of ketosis is that your blood sugar is stable and your insulin is low. This means that your body should not be giving off the feelings of hunger. With lowered insulin, the hormone ghrelin is also low and will not tell your brain that it needs to be fed first thing in the morning.

Usually, after a short adjustment period, many women neither crave or need to eat breakfast.

How Intermittent Fasting Can Slow Down Aging Process

One great benefit to intermittent fasting is that it can actually slow down the aging process. Mitochondria are structures in the cells that produce energy. They change in their shape in the response of energy demand. However, as we age, they lose the ability to do so. In a study that focused on mitochondria in the cells, there was evidence that they were able to retain 'youthfulness' longer by dietary restrictions such as intermittent fasting.

Chapter Three

The Lean Gain Method

Often, when people hear of the term "intermittent fasting" they also think if the term "lean gains." Lean gains are one of the programs that brought intermittent fasting to light in more recent years. Originally designed for rapid muscle building and fat loss, it has become a popular term in the dieting industry.

Lean gains is a dieting approach that basically takes three types of dieting and melts them all into one. The lean gain approach was created as an optimal solution to getting fit and having an efficient healthy diet. Basically, the lean gain method consists of intermittent fasting, usually the sixteen hours fast and the eight-hour feeding window; however, there is some debate on whether or not women benefit more from a fourteen hour fast with a ten-hour eating window. There is some variation depending on personal preference and need. It consists of weight training, classic lifts and squats, and all the typical strength training techniques.

Lean gains also consist of high protein diet on a daily basis while strength training days are high on carbs and low fat; nevertheless, the rest of the time is on moderate fat and low carbs. The lean gain approach is one that many people have heard of and associate with the term intermittent fasting. It was ultimately designed to help men get fit and ripped fast while using intermittent fasting as an aid and timed meals and calorie intake. In the lean gain method, it is recommended that you eat post workout or strength training. It is also recommended to perform strength training three times per week and there have been some decent results with the studies. Many subjects lost a significant amount of body fat while gaining significant muscle. Essentially, the lean gain approach tricks your body into thinking it is on a diet, while really you are just limiting the time that you are feeding and adjusting your caloric, fat, and carb intakes.

The lean gain method is one of the names that brought intermittent fasting to light and made it popular in recent culture. Like with all things that have to do with intermittent fasting, it is beneficial to many but not necessarily right for everyone. While women can certainly participate and have good results from the lean gains system and protocols, it was and always will be more targeted for men interested in strength training and fast results.

Most women engage in intermittent fasting by following one of two of the most popular protocols. There is the 'sixteen eight protocol'. The sixteen eight protocol is where you fast for sixteen hours and then have an eight hour feeding period. This is popular as it can be a way of life.

Getting Started With Intermittent Fasting

Most Common Fast Periods:

- Sixteen hours fast with an eight-hour feeding window
- Twelve and twelve-twelve hour fast, twelve-hour feeding window
- Fourteen and ten-fourteen hour fast, ten hour feeding period
- The twenty-four hour fast should be performed no more than two times per week

When jumping into the lifestyle of intermittent fasting, first establish a plan. Do your research and decide what fast is best for you. There will be a certain amount of trial and error. A good place to start is the sixteen hour fast with an eight-hour feeding window. Plan out what you are going to break your fast with ahead of time and have a time planned. It is best to do it on a day when you are busy and have plans, especially if you tend to be an emotional eater. Keeping busy will help with keeping you distracted and absent-mindedly eating. Have a stock of herbal teas and black coffee if you think you are going to have trouble your first day. Keep it in mind that it will get easier. It takes a few days for your body to adjust to the fasting lifestyle. But remember, it will adjust. Our bodies are well equipped for prolonged periods of fasting, it is just an adjustment period. It is also okay to not be successful immediately. There will be a trial and error and the standard fasting periods do not always work for everyone. It is okay to adjust your schedule to what better fits your needs, your lifestyle, your workout schedule, and your daily life in general. It is ok to adjust your fast and eating period as well.

While the sixteen and eight-fast and feeding period is easily the most common and can be safely used every day, it does not mean it is necessarily the best fit for you personally. If you start off with a sixteen-hour fast and find it is simply too much for you at first, start with a smaller window. Start with a twelve-hour fast and build up to where you want to be. Some women do better with a fourteen-hour fast and a ten-hour feeding window, and then some prefer a twenty-hour fast and a four-hour feeding window. Everyone is different and what is most important is what works for your schedule, lifestyle, comfort levels, and that ultimately gives you the best results with fasting.

Planning Your Meals After a Fast

Planning your post fast meals has a lot of room for customization. Finding the best solution for you can require some trial and error. Once you break your fast, it is important not to immediately inhale your food and continue eating nonstop through your fasting period. Eat something that is high in good fat and go from there. Many women find that in their feeding period they only eat two regular meals, while others eat three. Some prefer to just snack continuously through the feeding period. While you are still adjusting to intermittent fasting, it is not uncommon to feel ravenously hungry at first. This is part of why it is so important to break your fast slowly and with certain foods. When first getting started, one of the absolute most important tricks to success is having your day and meals planned out and then sticking to them. The more you have planned, the less likely you will be tempted with foods that do not go well with intermittent fasting. As with any diet change, you will be more successful with self-monitoring. Having a plan helps you to keep self-control better and you will be less likely to binge eat or impulse eat after coming out of your fasting state. When you are first adjusting is when this is most critical. You will be very hungry at first because it takes three to five days for your hormones to self-regulate. Once your insulin has naturally stabilized, ghrelin hormone will also adjust and begin telling you that you are hungry at your new meal times. The body likes routine and adjusting to fasting is simply teaching your body a new routine. Planning your meals and knowing what and when you are going to eat will drastically help with the adjustment period.

Breaking Your Fast

Care should be taken when breaking your fast, so you do not overwhelm your digestive system. It is important to not overeat right after you have completed your fast as this is a critical time for your digestive system. While in a fast, your metabolism is in a state of hormonal and physiological adaptions so in order to not disrupt and irritate the digestive tract, it is essential to follow some basic guidelines for ending your fast and entering your period of feeding time.

Guidelines While Breaking Your Fast

First, finding something to stimulate the digestive tract without releases insulin is ideal. Making a drink with lemon water, sea salt, two tablespoons of apple cider vinegar and cinnamon is a great way to wake up your digestive tract without upping your insulin, just hot lean water works as well. The citric acid from lemons helps to give the digestive enzymes a bit of a boost. The broth is another good fast breaker, especially bone broth. Bone broth is great for boosting collagen and easing your digestive tract back in. These starter beverages are especially useful for breaking a long fast; more than twenty hours when your gut is "asleep." For breaking a routine, twelve to sixteen-hour fast foods high in good fats are good for that. Avocados, a few eggs, or fish are all suitable for breaking a fast. The body will be in low-level ketosis and it will be more beneficial for it to transfer from burning its own fat to burning an ingested fat as opposed to a more complex carb to break down. When breaking a fast, the first meal should be relatively small. Under five hundred calories is ideal. This will help to re-acclimate your digestive system and adjust to food again.

The other common style of intermittent fasting is the twenty-four-hour protocol. This is where you do not eat for twenty-four hours. However, this protocol is slightly riskier, and you should not engage in it more than two days a week. When first beginning to fast, it is important to be mentally prepared for the challenge. At first, it will not come easily, and you will be fighting hunger. Essentially you are retraining your body that you do not need food as often as it thinks you do and this can take time.

The Four Main Types of Fasting

There are really four main types of fasting with different benefits. The most popular is intermittent fasting where you only eat for certain parts of the day. In a biological sense, all fasting is intermittent because you cannot simply live without calories and food. Fasting is more of a lifestyle approach and is certainly better for body composition.

The four types of fasting are intermittent fasting, prolonged fasting, liquid fasting, and dry fasting.

- Intermittent Fasting

Intermittent fasting is essentially what has been discussed this whole guide. Only feeding for certain parts of the day. As mentioned throughout, it has many benefits, the most popular being weight loss.

- Prolonged Fasting

There is also a form of fasting called prolonged fasting. This is a fast that lasts twenty-four to seventy-two hours. This is really only safe to do one to two times a month. It is good for cell rejuvenation. It is good to do on occasion as the body goes and hunts out the old and dying cells and feeds on them. This is called autophagy. Autophagy is basically how your body recycles cells. Prolonged fasting is good for longevity and fat burning. However, once you pass the forty-eight hours mark, there begins to have a few negative effects. So, if you choose to partake in a prolonged fast, twenty-four to forty-eight hours is the sweet spot. While this fast has its benefits, be sure to carefully monitor yourself throughout, and be sure to only follow this fasting protocol one to two times per month as using a prolonged fast too often, will create a calorie deficiency.

- The Liquid Fast

Metabolically speaking, the liquid fast is not a true fast. However, it is good for your digestive system. The liquid fast protocol is consisting of all liquids, and it is good to do one to two times a week. Liquid fasting is a good way to give the digestive system a break. Liquids are much easier to digest than solid foods. The liquid fast can consist of just about any liquid, jello type products, tea, and coffee. If you have a sensitive digestive system or irritable bowel, the liquid fast can be beneficial especially.

- The Dry-Fast

The dry fast is a rather extreme fast. To dry fast means to ingest nothing — no food and no water for an extended period of time, usually twenty-four hours. This fast is generally quite extreme and should only be done every three to six months. There are two different types of dry fasts. The soft fast, which is where you can still brush your teeth and the hard fast is where you do not. The dry fast does come with some risks; however, there are also benefits. It is extreme though and should only be done a few times a year. The dry fast is good if you have a lot of inflammation in your body. The lack of fluids pulls the water from the area that is inflamed. The dry fast is a good way to restart your digestive system and help your body to rid of retained water and extra edema. It should be used with great caution and great infrequency, however.

Getting It Right for You

Keep in mind that when you begin intermittent fasting, it is more of a lifestyle change than an actual diet and it is okay to not get it right a first. Finding out what works for you is a major part of being successful with intermittent fasting. Many women have found different schedules that work best for them. The other key point to keep in mind, is what is the rush? You do not need to figure out what best works for you on the first day. It is a good idea to take a little time and figure out what works best for you and your lifestyle before getting started. Find meal recipes and plan what you will eat ahead of time if you are unsure of things and feel you do not have enough support, try and find a friend to do it with. There are numerous online resources that offer great ideas, support, and advice. It is helpful to talk to your family doctor or a nutritionist before starting. They can potentially help you to tailor your diet and schedule to a system of eating and fasting that works for you the most adequately.

It is certainly a learning curve to adjust to such a lifestyle and it is important to cut yourself some slack. Try not to get frustrated if you see friends or other people have more success or different effects than you are having at first. Every woman is different, and every metabolism is different as well. It is always okay to give yourself time both to adjust and figure out your ideal program. A healthy lifestyle is not built in a day and there will be setbacks and annoyances along the way. One of the most important things to remember is that no matter how long it takes, or how difficult it is for you to adjust, you are still doing laps around the people that are not trying!

Special Advice for Overweight Women and Intermittent Fasting

Many people are drawn to intermittent fasting because of the weight loss benefits. While intermittent fasting is helpful and beneficial for weight loss, it is important to follow the correct protocols while starting out. Intermittent fasting is very beneficial for weight loss and one of the main reason women are interested in the lifestyle to start with. If you are overweight and want to participate in intermittent fasting for weight loss, it is best to thoroughly discuss with your doctor first. While some form of fasting can be beneficial to everyone, not all types or styles are right for every person. Discuss with your doctor your goals and what they believe the healthiest way to do it is.

Generally, overcoming hunger and emotional eating are the biggest hurdles. Many people are overweight because they tend to eat their feelings and emotions. Often, weight loss is difficult because women tend to turn to food for comfort. Intermittent fasting for weight loss does extremely well with a ketogenic type of diet. Combining the two gives excellent and fairly quick results. The other thing you will want to do if you are overweight and want to give intermittent fasting a try is to begin some form of exercise routine. This can start out as simply walking around the block or going for a bike ride. Doing some form of work out will help to allow fat to be burned more efficiently and will likely speed up the weight loss process. Many women see rapid weight loss when starting the intermittent fasting program while others see fewer results until combined with another traditional diet. Intermittent fasting has been so popular in the last few years because it has been so helpful to women losing weight.

Bypass or Weight Loss Surgery and Intermittent Fasting

It appears that there is a bit of controversy when it comes to whether or not intermittent fasting is a good idea after having weight loss surgery. Weight loss surgery is typically a gastric bypass; when the stomach is cut down to a small pocket and removed; a gastric sleeve where the stomach is contained to the approximate size of a banana or the lap band surgery where a band is placed around the stomach to make it smaller in size. Women that have had weight loss surgery have typically exhausted all diet options and needed the surgery to help them to lose the weight. Adding intermittent fasting in after a weight loss surgery can be tricky. Since the size of the stomach has been significantly reduced, calories and nutrients are not as easily absorbed. Since the intermittent fasting diet is meant to be over a feeding period, this often does not go well with bariatric surgery patients because they cannot physically eat enough calories to be healthy over the feeding period. If you are really interested in intermittent fasting after a weight loss surgery, then it is best to discuss with you

Type Two Diabetes

There are some recent studies that imply that intermittent fasting can be beneficial to individuals with type two diabetes. Fasting and diabetes have had a bit of controversy surrounding it but with some recent and updated information, there is some evidence that it can help regulate insulin and blood glucose levels. As mentioned above, intermittent fasting aids and allows the body hormones, like blood glucose and insulin, to naturally lower and regulate. Fasting for insulin regulation appeared to be especially helpful for women that have had trouble maintaining a diabetic diet seven days a week. It was suggested that if fasted for two twenty-four-hour periods in a week, that insulin and blood sugar levels stabilized in the diabetic patient. This new evidence can really help to improve the lives of diabetics everywhere. Regardless of the research, it is still best to consult with your regular doctor before using intermittent fasting as a diabetic.

Age

It appears that once you are over the age of eighteen, there are little negative effects of intermittent fasting in any healthy adult. In ancient times, intermittent fasting was practiced by all ages and they all seemed to benefit from the lifestyle. Granted, the times were different and they had little choice other than to fast due to having to hunt and gather food. There is very limited evidence that says age matters or is of significance to any healthy adult that wants to participate in intermittent fasting.

Children and Intermittent Fasting

There is a bit of medical controversy over whether children should participate in the intermittent fast. Most doctors agree that they should if the child is overweight or obese. Intermittent fasting can be very beneficial for weight loss in kids and teenagers. It can be a particularly hard adjustment, however. Kids tend to like to snack all day long and this can be difficult to break. It is important that the meals the child consumes are very nutrient dense and satisfying. Start with three meals a day in a twelve-hour window and then gradually attempt to bring it down to two meals a day. As long as the meals are heavy in good nutrients and good fats, most kids adapt with little trouble. Intermittent fasting is great for overweight kids and teens as well as athletic teens that are trying to build more muscle.

The negativity surrounding intermittent fasting in children mostly comes from a presumption that not eating will stunt growth. There is no scientific evidence that supports this claim and intermittent fasting is not typically recommended in small or young children anyway. Most research says that if the kid is overweight or trying to build muscle for sports, it is acceptable.

Long-Term and Negative Effects

There is little official research on long-term fasting effects, but what there is research on, shows that there are very few negative long-term effects on the body systems from intermittent fasting. Like the people who lived in stone ages and ancient times, fasting is normal, and our bodies are well equipped to handle it. However, it is important to remember that humans have not been cavemen for hundreds of years so it does take some adapting. While the majority of intermittent fasting has good health benefits, there are some negative effects that can occur. As with any diet or lifestyle change, it is important to be aware of all effects.

Feeling Full to the Point of Discomfort

This can occur when you have been fasting for a while. Your body gets used to having a reduced stomach size and when you first eat, you have to readjust to the amount of food you intake. With intermittent fasting, depending on your feeding window, you generally have to get some large dense meals to get the appropriate number of calories to be healthy especially right before you head into a fast. Getting used to having a full stomach for a few hours is simply something you will have to adjust too, to keep up the intermittent fasting program. The other unfortunate part of having to eat large nutrient dense meals is that it can add stress to your body and digestive systems.

Reliance on Caffeine

Another less than positive long-term effect is that you tend to get over addicted to caffeine. Mainly tea and coffee. Since coffee and tea are allowed, many women drink an abundance of it during a fast to stay energized. Unfortunately, a caffeine addiction comes with its own issues. This side effects can include anxiety, sleep deprivation, mood swings, and weight gain. For the average everyday caffeine addict, these side effects can eventually be problematic.

Athletic Performance Can Suffer

While it is generally good and effective to work out during a fast, you should not do extremely intense workouts, which means sometimes your athleticism can suffer. If you are on the two days a week for a twenty-four-hour schedule, you can still do heavy and intense weight training. There are studies that show without careful regulation, performance does eventually begin to suffer especially with cardio type exercise such as performance running.

Heartburn

Heartburn is a common occurrence during intermittent fasting, especially when first adjusting to the schedule and lifestyle. It often does eventually go away after five or six weeks but not always. The reason that heartburn occurs is that the body is confused by the abnormal eating pattern and lets off acid in the stomach periodically. When you suddenly change your eating pattern, the stomach tries to keep it on the schedule that it was on. Some people adjust quickly and some simply never adjust and have to deal with the heartburn. If it does persist, you can see your doctor, and antacids often help.

Headaches Throughout the Fast

Many people complain of headaches while fasting. There is some speculation about what causes them. Some say it is being in the state of ketosis, while others say it is simply dehydration and should go away with water intake. Likely, it is either or both that causes the head pain many people get every time they fast, unfortunately. You can play around with water intake and the amount of time you fast to try and ease some of the headaches.

Reoccurring Diarrhea

This is a surprisingly frequent occurrence with intermittent fasting. Many women get diarrhea of varying degrees while in a fast. This is typically due to the high fluid intake; a large amount of coffee, water, and tea. Often women have complained that the longer the fast, the more explosive the diarrhea is. Often it can be controlled with over the counter medications, but is an unpleasant side effect, regardless.

Long-Term Effects

Unfortunately, there is very limited research on the long-term effects of intermittent fasting on the body systems. There is evidence of increased lifespan and decreased aging, but the studies remain limited. Very few people stay in the intermittent lifestyle program for years on end. Historically, it was helpful and had great benefits for the people alive in the stone ages. In modern times, however, there simply is not enough research to back up the claims of zero negative long-term effects. This does not mean though that the potential negative effects of intermittent fasting actually exist. Overall, intermittent fasting is fairly safe to do for extended periods of time and gives many people great results for a variety of things.

Chapter Four

Evaluate Your Progress

Finding what works best for you is one of the biggest challenges when engaging in intermittent fasting. Intermittent fasting is about the time period you are eating in as opposed to what exactly you are eating. Even with that being said, it is important that you find eating habits that are suitable for your needs. Planning ahead when you are intermittent fasting is probably the most important piece of advice to help with success. Consider your habits and daily patterns and try to figure out ways to break up your bad habits. Do you like to get fast food on your way home? Try and plan ahead with a meal in the car. You will be surprised to see how quickly you can break a bad eating habit if you get out in front of it.

Finding Your Suitable Eating Portion

Portion control also plays an important role in the intermittent fasting way of life. It is important to monitor your portion size, especially when breaking a fast. While you are in a fasting state, your stomach constricts. When you begin to eat again, your stomach expands. If you do not manage your portion sizes when breaking a fast, your stomach will expand swiftly and your body will spend much more of your feeding period trying to insist it needs more food because your stomach has expanded.

Is Intermittent Fasting for You?

Before you jump headlong into the lifestyle of intermittent fasting, make sure that it is the proper choice for you personally. It is not a bad idea to consult with a doctor, nutritionist or dietician before beginning. Certain health risk factors make the intermittent fasting protocols unhealthy for certain individuals. While most women can certainly benefit, there are always exceptions and it is important to be a good fit for the diet to maintain good long-term health. Generally speaking, intermittent has health benefits that can be good for nearly everyone. There are certain situations that require you to proceed with caution when considering this type of eating pattern including pregnancy and nursing mothers, bariatric surgery patients, recovering from an eating disorder, and several other situations that should be approached with caution.

When to Stop Intermittent Fasting

Examples:

- Uncontrolled binge eating
- Metabolic disruption
- Lost menstrual cycles
- Early onset menopause
- Eating disorder relapse

There may be a time when you are engaging in the lifestyle of intermittent fasting that the protocols are no longer healthy for your lifestyle, body chemistry, mental health, or physical health. While it can be beneficial to most women, if you are finding you cannot control your binge eating, no matter what technique you try, it may be better to shorten your fasts. If you find your menstrual periods have become abnormal, your mood is too out of whack, or something simply just does not feel right, stop the lifestyle immediately. You do not want to do something that can permanently harm your health.

It is okay to take a step back and evaluate your goals and where you are in life. Not every dietary change is right for every woman and that is okay. You will know what diet plan is right for you, and if you really enjoy the benefits and lifestyle of intermittent fasting, you can talk to a doctor or nutritionist to determine which is the best and the safest way to proceed with intermittent fasting. There are cases where intermittent fasting simply is not right for. Knowing yourself and your body well enough to determine what feels right and what works best for you is important to any diet change or lifestyle. As was mentioned previously, it is okay to not get it right at first.

Pregnancy and Fasting

Pregnancy and fasting is a bit of uncharted territory when it comes down to it. Many doctors say to not do it, that it is not safe and that you really should be consuming an extra three to five hundred calories per day while other doctors say it is not such a big deal. The best advice that can ultimately be given on the subject is if you choose to continue intermittent fasting while pregnant, proceed with utmost caution.

If you are determined to continue the intermittent lifestyle during your pregnancy, consider a slightly easier schedule. Try and fourteen and ten-hour fast, or a twelve and twelve schedule. It is very important to get adequate nutrition throughout the pregnancy and to consume foods that are high in fiber. During the third trimester, it is often necessary to bump up your calorie intake a little to ensure you and the fetus are getting adequate nutrition the remainder of the pregnancy. If you are unsure if you should continue intermittent fasting or do not feel comfortable with it, it is wise to consult with a trusted family physician or your OBGYN to see what they think is safe for you and the fetus.

Breastfeeding is also uncharted territory when it comes down to intermittent fasting. Generally, it is discouraged because it can affect your milk production which could potentially harm your baby and slow the growth and progression. Overall it is best to avoid intermittent fasting while pregnant and nursing unless under very careful monitoring by a doctor.

Polycystic Ovarian Syndrome and Intermittent Fasting

Polycystic ovaries are a fairly common disease in women. This disease causes a hormone shift and can have any undesirable effects on women. Many women struggle with weight gain and difficulty losing weight as a side effect of the disease. While there are not very many studies about how intermittent fasting affects the disease, there is evidence that combining intermittent fasting with a keto diet significantly helped to regulate the hormones and made weight loss possible for polycystic ovarian syndrome patients. There does seem to be some potential hope with using intermittent fasting to help treat and maintain diseases like polycystic ovarian syndrome and other hormonal disorders. Time and additional research will tell us if intermittent fasting has a future in helping with this disease.

Overcoming Binging

A struggle many women live and fight with is binge eating. Binge eating is to eat an excessive amount, even though your body is no longer hungry, and it is generally a psychological habit. Binge eating actually is considered an eating disorder now. Binge eating is especially difficult for women that tend to be emotional eaters. Many women turn to food to control their feeling and this is both common and can be quite a challenge to overcome.

Emotional eating is when you literally want to eat whenever you have a strong feeling about something. Emotionally eating, or eating your feeling as some call it, very easily leads to binge eating. As with any bad habit, binge eating falls into the category of learning to break the habit. This is naturally much easier said than done. Many women have found distraction techniques as helpful to get control of their binge eating. Yoga, Pilates, and meditation are great ways to clear your mind and pull your focus away from emotionally eating.

Overcoming binging can be a real challenge and can take real work and willpower. It also is not always necessarily able to be broken immediately. It is important that you learn to listen to what your body is telling you instead of your emotions and this will help with overcoming binge eating. Many women need a professional psychologist or counselor to get over binge eating. Eating can also be an addiction and sometimes, advanced help is needed to break the unhealthy cycle of overeating. If you realize you are out of control with your binge eating, do not hesitate to get help, there are many good resources for support for women.

Adjusting Your Intermittent Fasting Schedule

Where there is intermittent fasting, there is also an adjustment period. The nice thing about intermittent fasting is that the schedule is determined by what works for you and your schedule. While the flexibility is convenient, it is still an adjustment for your body, for your mind, and your day to day activities. You will need to be cautious and really listen to what your body is telling you when you are starting out with intermittent fasting. Just because the sixteen hours fast with the eight-hour feeding window is popular, it does not mean it cannot be adjusted to fit your needs. Many women do better with a fourteen-hour fast and a ten-hour feeding window, however, sixteen is simply too much for them. This is the beauty of the fasting schedule; it is flexible and can be adjusted to your individual needs.

Chapter Five

How to Get the Best Out of Intermittent Fasting

Combining Intermittent Fasting with Exercise

Combining intermittent fasting with exercise is one of the best ways to get the most benefits and best results out of intermittent fasting. Combining work out with intermittent fasting and any other diet; like ketogenic, paleo or any other low carb type program will give you the best and the quickest results for weight loss. There are many ways to exercise including cardio, strength training or lifting, yoga, and Pilates. Any of these exercise styles and regiments can be beneficial and help with your ultimate goal of weight loss and a healthier life, but certain workouts have certain benefits. There are also time frames to exercise in during a fast that will help to optimize your results. Cardio is ideal for fat burning and strength training for building muscle. Yoga is great for core strength and certain yoga poses can actually help to regulate certain hormones. Nearly all exercise has benefits if you can find the time and the drive to make it part of your daily lifestyle.

When to Work Out

Most would consider the opportune time to work out to be in the middle of a fast. For example, let's say you started your fast at ten at night, working out after you wake up in the morning is considering an ideal time to work out or exercise as it is in the middle of your fast. You should still have ample energy as your body will not be expecting to be fed until later. Working out in the morning is also a great way to get going in the morning and is a natural way of waking up. Doing your work out in the middle or beginning of your fast is usually superior and you will feel better with better results as opposed to doing your work out toward the end of your fast.

When you are nearing the end of your fasting period, your body tends to be more fatigued and depleted of energy and you may find your work out less satisfying and beneficial. Some women choose to do their work out during their feeding period. This is generally not quite as beneficial as working out during the fast itself but is still better than not working out at all. Besides working out for strength, weight loss and overall health, exercise is proven to release mood-improving endorphins and boost energy. Overall, it is ideal to workout midway through your fast, but as mentioned, if you cannot work out mid fast or if your schedule does not allow it, anytime you can fit it in is better than not at all. Working out is quite important to help achieve the best possible results, so it is better to fit it in where you can than not at all!

Yoga and Pilates to Aid in Hormonal Balance

Many people have heard of the wonderful benefits of practicing yoga and Pilates. Yoga is relaxing, great for flexibility, and improving core and body strength. Yoga has been known to aid in pain relief and improve the mood, reset the mind and help with focus. Yoga is a great natural way to give your body a boost and to help relax and de-stress. Basically, yoga brings the three main elements together; exercise, breathing, and meditation. Pilates has a similar effect except it tends to focus more on lengthening and strengthening all the major and large muscle groups. Pilates particularly improves strength, body awareness, and balance. What is less known about Pilates and yoga is that it can actually help to stabilize and regulate the body's hormones with certain poses. The yoga poses can subtly pressurize and depressurize certain glands of the body. These minor compressions and decompressions can help to regulate hormonal secretions. Therefore, certain yoga poses can help to balance and stimulate certain endocrine functions. Many common negative feelings can be attributed to a hormonal imbalance. Feelings like being constantly tired, low self-esteem, anxiety, and emotional eating with a slow metabolism can all possible be effects of a hormonal imbalance in women.

A few of even the most basic yoga poses can help with hormone regulation. An easy pose that can have a big effect is the 'rabbit pose' also known as the Sasangasana pose. This is a beginner pose that nearly anyone can do that works to stimulate the thyroid gland. The thyroid gland is on your neck and is a horn responsible for secreting growth regulating hormones and metabolic function. To get into this yoga pose, start by sitting on your heels in 'hero pose' (sitting on your legs in a kneeling position with shins and top of feet on the floor, hands resting calmly on knees) then bring your arms back and grab onto your foot soles. Bring your chin to your chest and round your back and body forward, folding your body at the pelvis. When doing this, your head should come down towards the floor and your forehead should touch your knees. Bring your hips up a small amount as the top of your head touches the floor. Inhale five deeps breathes as you comfortably hold this position, then go back into your hero pose. Do this several times for the best effect.

The cobra pose, also known as 'Bhujangasana' is another simple yet effective pose that is good for hormone regulation. Specifically, the cobra pose is good for massaging the adrenal glands. Helping the adrenal gland function better can aid in helping your body to better fight stress and let go of tension easier. Start the cobra pose by lying flat on your belly with legs together and your hands on the floor even with your shoulders. Start with your forehead resting flat on the floor. Then simply lift your head and chest upward, lengthening your spine and stretching your core. Take several deep breaths, inhaling and exhaling slowly for several seconds and then lower yourself back to the ground. Do this pose several times and take a few minutes to really appreciate and enjoy the feeling of the cobra pose and its benefits.

The third simple, yet effective yoga pose for hormone regulation is the camel pose, also known as 'Ustrasana'. The camel pose has quite a large variety of known advantages and benefits. One of them being, of course, to aid in the regulation of hormones. As the pose is being held, it helps to stimulate the internal organs and structures especially in the neck and shoulder regions of the body. As was stated earlier, this is where the thyroids glands are located, and they appear to really like the benefits of the camel pose. To begin the camel pose, start with a kneeling position. Keep your knees at the same width apart as your pelvis. Bring your thighs in towards each other and bring your pelvis forward and up towards the torso. Meanwhile, be sure you are keeping your shins and feet firmly pressed to the ground. Take your hand to the back of your hips with your palms toward your body. Push down on your tailbone area with your palms as you push your thighs back to compensate your body moving forward. Then take a big deep breathe as your shoulder blades move in the direction of your ribs. Lean backward a little bit and relax your torso and rib areas as you relax and pull your chest away from your hips. Take your hands down to your heels and move your arms out. Try and hold the position for thirty to forty-five seconds before bringing up your upper body and returning to the original position. Perform the position several times to really get the best effects and hormone affecting benefits.

The reason that yoga and Pilates can aid in being successful on your intermittent fasting journey is that it can help to control cravings and hunger, it is good exercise, and most importantly, it helps with the hormonal balancing. A large part of what makes intermittent fasting beneficial and why women are seeing such great results with it is that it is helping to naturally regulate the body's hormones to better acclimate it to a faster and more efficient metabolism. So while yoga has great benefits for the mind, body, and soul, it is also great for natural hormonal regulation!

Cardio — Running, Cycling, and Swimming to Help with Intermittent Fasting Results

There was a myth going around for a while that doing cardio on an empty stomach can help with losing the 'stubborn' fat. This is false. Doing fasted cardio is actually what helps to lose those stubborn fat places. To define what exactly cardiovascular exercise is, it is an aerobic exercise that uses oxygen to meet the demands of energy during exercising. Examples of cardio workouts are swimming, running, cycling — basically any aerobic type activity. This basically means it is an exercise that specifically works the heart, the lungs, and that oxygen intake is required to participate in.

To break it all down, cardio done in a fed state is not quite as effective as cardio performed in a fasted state. The difference between an empty stomach and a fasted state is essentially when you do your cardio. If you do your cardio in your feeding window, you are not in the fasted state of lowered insulin and blood sugar and your body is working on processing the foods you have been feeding it in your eating window. While generally any exercise burns energy and helps you to lose weight no matter what your insulin levels are at, there are some pretty specific benefits of doing your cardio in a fasted state. One of the subtle benefits of doing cardio in a fasted state is that lipolysis and fat oxidation rates are increased.

Basically, lipolysis is the breaking down of fat cells by the body to use as energy. Essentially, this means to enter a fat burning state. Fat oxidation simply means the burning of this energy by the cells. So cardio exercise helps the body to break down and burn fat stores easier in a fasted state. The claims of fasted cardio helping with 'stubborn belly fat' stem from the studies that show increased blood flow to the stomach and abdominal reasons in the state of a fast. With minimal blood flow to a certain area or region of the body, it means less fat burning chemicals and therefore there is a less fat loss to certain areas of the body with less blood flow.

Fasted cardio is a bit of a double-edged sword in the sense that there are a few downsides to it. There is some evidence that fasted cardio can cause some muscle breakdown as well. While this generally is not catastrophic or really, all that significant, it can have an effect. This is not ideal because if you break down enough muscle too quickly. Your body will not be able to keep up with the repairs required to build more muscle and could eventually actually lead to muscle loss. Ultimately fasted cardio to aid with weight loss and overall health is more beneficial than not. But as mentioned, it does come with a couple of risks and should be used with care and caution. Cardio is generally great for cardiac health and stamina, regardless of what diet plan or routine you are on.

Strength Training and Intermittent Fasting

Strength training combined with intermittent fasting and healthy eating can provide some truly great results. Strength training, also known as weight lifting or resistance training is anaerobic exercise based off using resistance to cause muscle contraction, which in turn builds muscle, improves anaerobic endurance and enlarges the size of the skeletal muscles.

Many people believe that strength training is more beneficial than cardio of exercise when combining it with intermittent fasting. The theory is that it is an ideal way to maintain lean body mass is by intermittent fasting and strength training regularly as well as following a high protein low carb diet. Many women see great results combining these things.

Resistance training is more for building muscle than burning fat but is also excellent for maintaining the lean body mass. Doing strength training during the fasted state is typically giving the best results. If you do resistance training during a feeding period, keep in mind that your body is working on other things like digesting food and re-acclimating to the feeding period. Many women have said they have more energy and feel they have more effective workouts when performing their resistance training during a fast, as they are hyper-focused on the task at hand. Ultimately, strength training is an excellent addition to the intermittent fasting lifestyle and many women are achieving excellent results.

Meditation and Mindfulness

Meditation can be an excellent tool for focus, clearing the mind and aiding in success with any lifestyle change, especially intermittent fasting. It is an ancient technique that helps to focus and clear the mind. Meditation actually changes the structure of the brain and allows it to be clear and promote simple clear thoughts. It can give you almost superhuman abilities like being able to keep a calm clear head in a high-pressure situation and use the power of the mind to your advantage.

In the last ten years, scientists have discovered that every time we think or learn something, new a neuro connection appears in the brain. The neuro connections we use the most frequently, like a habit or routine, grow stronger with each use and weaker over time they are not in use until they eventually disappear. This is why certain habits are completely automatic. These are the same reasons that meditation is exceptionally useful for starting and using intermittent fasting. It helps to reinforce the habits necessary to be successful and to embed them in the brain. When you first begin to fast, it is often said how difficult the first few days are. Meditation can really help to clear the mind and allow you to focus on the challenge at hand. Usually, this is overcoming your hunger. Many women use meditation to get through the first stages of hunger and it really helps to reduce their stress, hanger, and hanxiety while your body adjusts to you first several fasting periods.

When and if you first decide to give meditation a try, there are several steps and techniques that you can follow to have a successful meditation. Start with finding a quiet atmosphere where you are either alone or a place that you are able to relax and clear your mind. Choose loose fitting and comfortable clothes for your meditation session, it is important to be comfortable and relaxed. Keep in mind that you will need to sit the whole time so wear something that is comfortable for that. Doing pre-meditating yoga and or stretches is recommended especially focusing on the back and neck as these are the places that we tend to hold stress in the most. Once you have found a place, outfit and time that is suitable for your meditation you can begin. A basic position is either sitting cross-legged or in the 'lotus' position which is cross-legged with the soles of your feet pointing upward. If you have difficulty with either of these positions, just sit as comfortably as you can. Begin by closing your eyes and focusing on your breathing, focus on your inspirations and expirations while attempting to let your other thoughts fall away. Do not try to control your breathing and try not to focus on anything else. When first starting out, only meditate for five to seven minutes a day.

When you are incorporating meditation with intermittent fasting, begin doing it when you start to feel initial pangs of hunger that you feel you cannot ignore. After you meditate, you should feel calm and relaxed and with luck, it will help to distract you from your hunger. It is ideal to meditate at the same time every day. Your body likes routine and it will begin to expect meditation at a certain time. People that are experienced in meditation can do it for up to twenty to thirty minutes a day. Practicing meditation is a great way to help you to overcome hunger, focus on your daily important tasks, and prepare your mind for a fast. There are many great resources available for free online to help you with practicing meditation.

Combining Intermittent Fasting with Other Diets

Since intermittent fasting is not really a diet, it is a pattern of feeding and fasting, and many women combine it with other diet plans. Intermittent fasting goes along great with other diets and women are getting great results. Intermittent fasting is compatible with many diets because it is adjustable and based less off of what is being consumed and more of when food is being consumed. The most popular diets that intermittent fasting is combined with is the ketogenic diet, the gluten-free diet, the paleo diet, and a vegan diet.

Combining Intermittent Fasting with a Ketogenic Diet

As many people already know, ketogenic diets have become exceptionally popular in the past several years. Combining both a keto diet and an intermittent fasting lifestyle is probably the best, quickest, and most effective way to lose weight. The keto diet is incredibly popular because it is so effective, especially in women. The keto diet is based on a high fat, low carb, and moderate protein type of protocol. Combining a keto diet with intermittent fasting can be extremely beneficial and productive, especially for weight loss and overall health.

The theory behind a ketogenic diet is that you achieve ketosis which is a stable level of blood sugar. The keto diet is based on high fat because fat is one of the first sources of fuel that your body converts into energy when consumed. By feeding your body high in healthy fat foods, it helps it to be more efficient in the breakdown. There are numerous benefits to combining intermittent fasting with a ketogenic diet; you will get very few cravings for starters. One of the desirable effects of the ketogenic diet is that it is exceptional at stabilizing blood sugar. Since keto is fat based, you will not get spikes in your blood sugar and therefore your insulin will not rise and give you food cravings. A ketogenic diet already is known for suppressing hunger.

When you are on a ketogenic diet, it encourages the liver to produce more keynotes. The ketones get into your bloodstream and the cells use them as fuel. Ketones also are known for suppressing ghrelin, the body's hormone that tells you when to eat. With the ketogenic diet already suppressing your hunger, fasting comes significantly easier and allows you to fast in longer windows and get the benefits of a longer fast.

Fat loss is another excellent benefit to combining the two diets. Both intermittent fasting and the keto diet increase fat loss, even without calorie restriction. Together the two eating styles create a superhuman fat burning machine. Many women drop weight swiftly and because the ghrelin hormone has already been suppressed, you do not feel nearly as deprived and hungry as you would with a traditional diet plan.

Ketosis

When hearing about a ketogenic diet, the term ketosis also come up. At one point, it was thought that being in a state of ketosis was bad for you. However, the ketogenic diet is based on being in a state of ketosis, this is actually the goal. Ketosis is a state in which the metabolism achieved where there are heightened ketones in the bloodstream and body tissues. It is a state of naturally lowered insulin. Ketones are water-soluble protein bodies that are produced by the liver from fatty acids during periods of low food intake or carb restricted diets. Ketosis helps the body to transition to a state of fat burning. When in ketosis, you will unlikely feel very hungry because your insulin is naturally lowered. Ketosis is the goal for following a ketogenic diet as it is the state in which the body is burning stored fat. In the fat burning state is when the most weight loss occurs.

Keto flu

Many women that live a keto lifestyle are familiar with the term 'keto flu.' This is basically your body's reaction to taking away its carbs. When you stop your carb intake, your body is no longer using carbs as its primary fuel source. When you are no longer using carbs for fuel, your body enters a state of ketosis, which is when it switches to burning fat. The symptoms come from your body adjusting to running off ketones. Ketones are what your liver produces during periods of fasting or starvation and are by-products of fat breakdown.

Many people really struggle with the lack of carbs and show symptoms within just a day or two. Symptoms can range in severity, some being mild to non-existent and others lasting longer. The average length of keto flu is about a week. Symptoms include nausea, vomiting, constipation, poor concentration, lack of energy, stomach pain, dizziness, weakness, irritability, muscle soreness, sugar cravings, and difficulties sleeping. To combat the keto flu, it is important to stay well hydrated and get enough sleep. Other ways to help combat the keto flu include getting enough electrolytes, avoiding excessive exercise, avoiding ambient light, and getting enough fat in your diet.

Taking good care of yourself during the first few days of transitioning to keto and fasting is essential in staying healthy. Be sure to plan your eating and meals ahead of time. Many women do a slow step down from carbs instead of going cold turkey to help avoid the keto flu. Cutting out just a few carbs each day and adding more fat is a common technique to adjust the body to the change. You still may get symptoms of the keto flu, but it may help them be less severe. It is also a good idea to switch either to keto or intermittent fasting first. Sometimes doing them both together can be too much stress on your body at once. Adapting to intermittent fasting first will help with one change at a time. Not everyone gets the keto flu, but do not be alarmed if you do.

As with most unpleasant things, it will pass, and you can hurry it along with supportive care for yourself.

Combining Intermittent Fasting with a Vegan Diet

Combining intermittent fasting with a vegan diet can be a greater challenge as vegan or plant-based food does not have healthy fats as readily available as animal-based foods. Having said that, it is not impossible and can still be conducive with the lifestyle of intermittent fasting. Basically, the difference between eating a regular diet and eating a vegan diet is that vegans do not eat any animal-based foods. They strictly eat plant-based foods and fruits, vegetables and substitutes like tofu etc. What makes combining veganism with intermittent fasting difficult the lack of natural fats available. When your body enters a fat burning state, it is more difficult to break a fast without any animal-based product. It is not impossible though and many vegans have had luck with it. Like with any diet, there are loopholes and ways to make it work with your lifestyle. Many vegans simply just have to eat more carbs. Nuts and seeds are good sources of protein and fat and are popular in a vegan diet in general.

Ultimately, since intermittent fasting is not exactly a diet as opposed to a pattern of eating, you technically do not need to change and supplement the vegan diet. While veganism can have excellent health benefits, it can be a struggle to get all the proper nutrition without an animal-based diet. The human body was designed to break down and ingest animal-based fats and food so training it to live off of plant-based foods can be a challenge. Most vegans will need to supplement with vitamins and minerals to meet all the health needs. Ultimately though, it is possible to live and remain healthy on a vegan diet along with engaging in intermittent fasting.

Humans are omnivores and should be able to adequately adjust to sole plant-based diets as long as they are properly supplemented. When beginning intermittent fasting with your vegan lifestyle, it is always a good idea to get advice or consult with your regular physician to find out the best and healthiest ways to safely participate.

Combining with a Paleo Diet

Combining intermittent fasting with a paleo diet is about as simple as you can get. Basically, a paleo diet is a diet based off what food was consumed during the stone ages and ancient times. When there were no stores, supermarkets, delis, and fast food restaurants, what was left? There were plants, meats, berries, vegetables, and whatever food could be hunted, picked, made or gathered.

Back in stone age times, when paleo eating was the only available way of life, intermittent fasting was already part of the lifestyle. It was part of life because food just was not always available. So, paleo diets are quite simple and go well with intermittent fasting. If you were to pretend you were living in ancient-paleo times, you would already be participating in intermittent fasting because that was a natural part of life in those days. Depending on where you lived, there were winters and food was not always available to be picked and gathered. Animals moved south, and hunting became scarce. So, what did you do when there was no food to be found? You simply did not eat, and your body adapted until you could.

In recent popular culture, the paleo diet has been enormously helpful in helping women with weight-loss and engaging in a natural basic diet by simply cutting out process food, carbs, and anything with preservatives. The paleo diet strips it all down to the basics of the human needs for food. A diet that simply involves protein, fruits, and vegetables. Combining this diet with intermittent fasting and some regular exercise can and will result in excellent results as far as feeling better and more energized and with weight loss.

The Gluten-Free Diet and Intermittent Fasting

Many people have seen the effects and benefits of going gluten-free. People with digestive and stomach issues often change to gluten-free. Gluten-free goes just as well with intermittent fasting as any other diet. It is important to keep an eye on your caloric intake as gluten-free diets often are carb free as well. Gluten-free diets tend to have a lot of foods that contain a lot of flour, so watch out for the carb count when eating gluten-free. Many women that are gluten-free already have good grasps of what goes well with their diet and where they can find foods that work for them. Adding in the timed fasting is just one step further that can take you closer to your goals and help to lead to a better and healthier life.

Essential Oils to Help with Intermittent Fasting and Weight Loss

Essential oils are a rapidly growing fad and are useful for many different ailments and can provide support for multiple body systems. While the use of essential oils is controversial in their effectiveness, many women swear by them and there is some evidence they can help with weight loss as well as provide immune support as well as mental health support. The route in which to use essential oils is varied. They can be used in a diffuser, inhaled in an inhaler, rubbed on the skin, made into body wraps, burned in candles, and many more options. They work both topically and aromatically. There are five specific essential oils geared toward weight loss as well as many that help with psychological challenges.

Grapefruit Essential Oils

Grapefruit essential oils contain d-limonene, a chemical that increases the rate of the metabolism because it induces lipolysis or the breakdown of fat cells. Grapefruit essential oils also help to fight cellulite in women. Grapefruit essential oils work best as a massage oil or bath salt. Grapefruit essential oils can be used daily for best results.

Peppermint Essential Oils

Peppermint is a great oil for energy and can really help to stifle cravings. It is refreshing to smell and has positive effects when inhaled; it is a natural bronchodilator and helps improve oxygen flow. Peppermint essential oils work best when inhaled directly. Put it in a diffuser for twenty minutes a day or put several drops onto a cloth or handkerchief and inhale directly for best results.

Lemon Essential Oils

Lemon smells fantastic and is quite useful in helping to block out thoughts of greasy foods and sugar. It has properties that help to improve energy and helps to increase your mood. Lemon essential oils are great for right before a workout. It works best in a diffuser for fifteen to twenty minutes.

Rosemary Essential Oils

Rosemary has an herbal, refreshing type smell and can really help in suppressing the appetite. Rosemary can help with water retention and surpass craving as well as help with cellulite prevention. Give it a sniff when you are struggling with a certain food craving. It is also a great massage oil and is effective as a bath salt. Rosemary has other health benefits as well and can even help with menstrual-related bloating.

Ginger Essential Oils

Ginger is a powerful detox aid. Ginger has detoxifying effects that are quite helpful with purging the body and mind of cravings and toxins. Ginger also helps to stimulate the lymph nodes, and it helps to stimulate blood flow and goes great in a bath! Many women mix with coconut oil and use topically. Ginger should be used with some caution as it is a "hot" oil and can cause the feelings of burning. Mixing four to five drops of ginger essential oil and two to three tablespoons of coconut oil and adding it to your bath is a great way to reap the benefits of ginger!

Lavender Essential Oils

Lavender is perhaps the most popular and well-known essential oil. Probably because it has such a diverse range of uses and effects. Lavender's best known for its calming properties. These are especially useful for when and if you experience 'hanger' or anxiety during a fast. Lavender helps to calm the irritability. Lavender is also a good sleep aid and can be used in a variety of forms. It can be applied topically, inhaled or ingested.

While essential oils certainly are not for everyone, they can and do help many women to overcome struggles both with intermittent fasting and wit weight loss in general. Sometimes, a sniff of the right oil is all you need to get over the hurdle at hand, whether it is to maintain a fast or get past a craving. The first few days of a fast or diet are always the most difficult and any support you can get is usually worth considering. They certainly have a place in a healthy life if you are willing to give them a try.

The Buddy System

Having a friend to endeavor into the intermittent fasting lifestyle with can make all the difference. For any life change, it is important to have a strong support system, you want to have someone to bounce off ideas, questions, and concerns with. Ask your friends and family if they are interested in a healthier lifestyle and find someone to do it with you. If no one you know personally is interested, there are various great blogs, discussion groups, and social media pages specifically for people that want to participate in the intermittent fasting and healthy eating lifestyle. Having a friend or support system to lean on especially when getting through your first few fast where your body is still adjusting to the new pattern can really make all the difference in success. There are also podcasts and talk shows that have great info about personal struggles and successes while intermittently fasting. Be sure to have a solid support system before beginning intermittent fasting.

Supplements and Vitamins to Aid in Fasting

Getting adequate vitamins and proper nutrition is absolutely vital while doing the intermittent fasting lifestyle. It is especially important because intermittent fasting is essentially forcing your body into a state of fat burning. In a state of fat burning, you are also in ketosis typically. Taking supplemental vitamins may be necessary during your fasting periods, especially if you are engaging in a long-term fast. Most multivitamins will due, but it is important to know what is in them and what they should contain to aid with your fast.

Sodium and Potassium

Levels of ketones in the bloodstream rise during your periods of fasting which cause your body to signal a flushing response. This quickly depletes the stores of potassium and sodium. It can cause fatigue, low energy, and the feeling of being lightheaded. These minerals are very important for ketogenesis and without them, the body really must work and struggle to access the stores of fat.

Magnesium

Magnesium is a body mineral that regulates several vital body functions. Magnesium helps to regulate nerve and blood pressure and is easily and swiftly depleted in the period of fasting. Low magnesium is what can cause the feeling of brain fogginess or muscle cramps during a fasting period.

B-Complex Vitamins

B-complex vitamin, which includes riboflavin, niacin, thiamine, and biotin are vitamins that aid the body in absorbing nutrients. B-complex vitamins do not get flushed out of the body in the same way sodium, potassium, and magnesium does during the state of ketosis. However, there are a large number of women that are chronically low or have B-complex vitamin deficiencies.

Vitamin D

Vitamin D is a very common deficiency amongst both men and women. Vitamin D is rather difficult to obtain through food intake and is acquired naturally through sunlight. Vitamin D is vital to both immune health and bone density. Vitamin D helps the use nutrients that are critical to body functions and helps allow the nutrients to function, magnesium being one of them.

Chromium

Chromium is not as common in your everyday multivitamin but there has been some research that shows it can be a culprit that mitigates hunger. This can be problematic as it may force you to end your fast earlier than planned or expected due to the hunger pangs.

Beta-Hydroxybutyrate or BHB

Many women who intermittently fast also take a BHB supplement as well, these are also known as exogenous ketones. This means ketones that are not produced by the body. One of the three ketone bodies is BHB. Ketone bodies are what is naturally produced by the liver when you are in a state of ketosis. If broken down to the cellular level, the human body needs BHB to access and adequately use the fat stores for energy. Using a BHB supplement during a fast helps to ensure that the body will have the necessary levels of BHB in the bloodstream. Having the proper levels of BHB in the bloodstream will help to facilitate the metabolizing of fat into energy.

Branched Chain Amino Acids

Branched-chain amino acids are amino acids that produce the same important amino acids that are found in protein. These amino acids allow the body to not only help build muscle but also to help sustain it. The downside to Branch Chain Amino Acid supplements is that they do contain a few calories, something around six calories per gram and could potentially disrupt a fast to a certain extent. Most people take Branch Chain Amino Acid supplements when they are working on strength training and building muscle as part of their daily routine. While many people have good positive effects with this supplement and experience no negative impact, this is not always the case and if having a strictly calorie free fast is important to you personally, this may be a supplement to avoid.

Water (H2O)

Drinking water is absolutely vital to any and all diets and fasts. This cannot be stressed enough. Lack of hydration is often the biggest factor in nearly all negative side effects to any fast. Body organs and tissues including the brain depend and utilize water to maintain the proper levels of nutrients, vitamins, and minerals. Dehydration has a wide variety of symptoms and can quickly lead to fatigue, irritability, dizziness, confusion, headache, and many other symptoms and feelings of discomfort. Maintaining proper hydration throughout a fast is important and allows any supplemental vitamins to work better.

Ultimately, taking a good multivitamin during a fast can significantly help your body systems out and help your fast be just a little bit easier.

Taking proper supplementation can aid in muscle building and help to improve the positive benefits of the fasting lifestyle. Choose a vitamin that contains what was just covered and you will be able to reap the benefits a little bit easier.

Alcohol and Intermittent Fasting

Many women enjoy having a beer or margarita after a long day, socially, or just for fun. The trouble with drinking while fasting is that there are calories in an alcoholic drink. Depending on what hours you are eating and fasting, you will need to plan to drink only during feeding periods. Drinking will break a fast. As far as healthier options with alcohol, low-calorie drinks are ideal, beer tends to be high in carbs. There are various recipes for 'skinny' margaritas and martinis. There are even low carb beers available. The most important things to remember with all intermittent fasting protocols is that when you eat is always more important than what you eat. Keeping yourself well hydrated is important to any diet, but it is especially important to an intermittent fasting diet plan which makes it even more important if you choose to drink while in an intermittent fasting program.

Pop or Soda and Intermittent Fasting

Drinking pop on a fast will without a doubt bring your fast to a screeching halt. Pop is high in sugar and chemicals that your body can really struggle with breaking down. Even diet pops are not particularly good. They are hard on the digestive system and can be corrosive to the gut lining. If you are a pop-acholic, it may be best to consider giving it up or at the very least switching to diet pop. Try and avoid even diet pop during a fast and especially regular pop as it will immediately reverse to the state of ketosis. Many women found they had weight losses simply by cutting pop out of their daily diet.

Chapter Six

While it has been mentioned several times that intermittent fasting is more of a lifestyle as opposed to a diet, there are certain recipes and eating patterns that can aid in intermittent fasting. Certain meals and eating patterns can help to bring out and encourage the benefits of intermittent fasting. Below are several examples that are simple and easy to make that work nicely with an intermittent fasting program. Several of the recipes are both keto-based and gluten-free. There are lots of great options for healthy delicious meals that are easy to prepare!

Three Simple and Easy Recipes for Breakfast

The Caprese Omelet — Healthy and Low-Carb

The healthy, low carb Caprese Omelet is easy and a good vegetarian option (not vegan though).

It can be made in just minutes and is an excellent filler. It is great with either store bought or homemade pesto.

- Three large eggs
- One tbsp. of butter or <u>ghee</u>
- One-third of a cup of cherry tomatoes, cut in half
- Two slices fresh mozzarella cheese
- Three to six basil leaves, chopped up well
- One heaped tbsp. grated parmesan cheese
- One tbsp. pesto
- Sea salt and pepper, or to taste
- Additional Option: One tsp. of balsamic vinegar and one tbsp. extra virgin olive oil to drizzle on top of the omelet

The Instructions: Combine ingredients together in a bowl, be sure to mix well. Use a medium pan and add a little butter and melt. Pour mixture in and heat until the egg is cooked on one side. Then fold omelet in half and cook both sides until done. Drizzle balsamic vinegar and olive oil if desired.

The Super Electrolyte Smoothie and Cereal

This smoothie and cereal are a great breakfast, snack, or evening meal that is both delicious, simple to make, and great for keeping yourself on a healthy track. While these are keto diet based, they are still great breakfast options. They are both quick and easy to prepare with easy to find ingredients.

Super Electrolyte Smoothie:

- One-half of a large avocado or three and a half ounces
- One-half of a cup of coconut milk such as Aroy-D or four fluid ounces
- One-third of a cup of frozen mixed berries or one and a half ounces
- One and a half cups unsweetened almond milk or cashew milk or twelve fluid ounces
- One tbsp. raw cacao powder or a quarter of an ounce
- One-fourth of a tsp. cinnamon
- One-fourth of a tsp. vanilla bean powder
- Two tbsp. of collagen powder or half an ounce

The Instructions: Blend well in a blender until smooth and pourable, then pour into a glass to enjoy.

Super Cereal (Keto-Based)

- One-fourth of a cup flaked almonds or twenty-three grams
- One-fourth of a cup unsweetened flaked coconut or fifteen grams
- One-fourth of a tsp. of cinnamon powder

- One tsp. of virgin coconut oil
- Toppings:
  - Two tbsp. of cacao nibs or one ounce
  - Two tbsp. of hemp seeds or three-quarters of an ounce
  - Optional: Fresh or frozen berries for the top

The Instructions: Add to a bowl and add fresh or frozen berries to the top.

Low-Carb Porridge – Anti-Inflammatory

This is a great warm breakfast, especially for the winter. It is unique because it contains some beneficial supplements such as turmeric (a spice that helps our body adapt to changes), and bee pollen (bee pollen has immune boosting properties and natural anti-inflammatory properties). If you are dealing with any kind of chronic pain or inflammation, this is an ideal meal for you.

- Two tbsp. of hemp seeds
- One-fourth of a cup of walnut or pecan halves
- One-fourth of a cup of unsweetened toasted coconut
- Two tbsp. of whole chia seeds
- Three-fourths of a cup of unsweetened almond milk
- One-fourth of a cup of coconut milk
- One-fourth of a cup of almond butter, preferably roasted
- One tbsp. extra virgin coconut oil or MCT oil or fifteen milliliters
- One-fourth to one half of a cup of ground turmeric or one half to one tsp. freshly grated turmeric
- One tsp. bee pollen or one-half tsp. cinnamon or one-half tsp. vanilla powder
- Pinch ground black pepper (significantly helps to improves turmeric absorption in the bloodstream)

- Optional: Two tbsp. Erythritol or Swerve or five to ten drops liquid stevia (NuNaturals or Sweet Leaf brands are ideal brands to use for this recipe)

Three Simple and Easy Recipes for Lunch

The Five-Minute Quick and Healthy Tuna Salad

This meal is easy to make and is full of superfoods, high in the good fats, and protein. This is ideal for lunch, after a workout, or for coming out of a fast. Tuna is a great lean protein and eggs are a good fat blast. Enjoy this tuna salad for lunch or for dinner.

- One-fourth of a cup of mayonnaise - Paleo mayonnaise is preferred
- One tbsp. of lemon juice or fifteen milliliters
- Two tbsp. of olive oil- extra virgin
- One tbsp. parsley or chives- chopped
- One-fourth of a tsp. each pepper and salt, or to taste
- One medium head of romaine lettuce
- One-half of a sliced small yellow or red onion
- One medium cucumber or four to five gherkins
- Eight sliced large olives
- One drained jar of tuna- large
- Four hard-boiled eggs- large

The Instructions: Combine the mayonnaise, parsley, onion, lemon juice, olive oil, and tuna in a bowl and mix well. Use the head of lettuce to make a lettuce bed and add tuna mixture to the top. Add the sliced hard-boiled eggs, olives, and cucumbers to the top. Serve and enjoy!

The All-Day Mexican Salad Bowl

This simple, delicious, and easy to make Mexican recipe is quick and packed full of healthy fats. This Mexican bowl is a great choice for helping to break a fast as it high in healthy fats that will help to keep your insulin levels stable. This Mexican bowl is quick and ideal for any time of the day!

- Two Mexican chorizo sausages
- Two gluten-free Italian style sausages
- One-half of a jalapeno pepper
- One tbsp. of fresh oregano or one tsp. dried oregano
- One small yellow onion, diced
- One-half of a cup of halved cherry tomatoes
- One-half of a red bell pepper, chopped well
- One medium spring onion, sliced well
- One tbsp. extra virgin olive oil or fifteen milliliters
- One-fourth of a tsp. of coconut aminos
- One tsp. of fresh lime juice
- One tbsp. of chopped and fresh coriander
- Two large eggs
- One-half of a large avocado, sliced
- One-fourth of a tsp. of paprika
- Salt and pepper to taste

Instructions: Cook sausage separately and add to salad, combine all ingredient, and enjoy!

Three Simple and Easy Recipes for Dinner

Green Chicken Chile Cauliflower Casserole

This is a relatively simple and quick dish to make that is both great for a keto diet and can be adapted to a gluten-free diet as well.

- One pound or four hundred and fifty grams of ground beef, turkey, chicken, or pork (chicken is most commonly used and the easiest)
- Two tablespoons butter

- Three-fourths of a cup of chopped onion
- Three-fourths of a cup of a chopped celery stalk
- Two and a half cups of cauliflower rice
- One cup of shredded Monterrey Jack cheese, or mozzarella cheese
- One cup of shredded sharp cheddar cheese
- One-half of a cup of chicken or vegetable broth
- Four ounces of canned green chiles - be sure to drain
- One-half of a cup of sour cream, full-fat variety
- One-half of a teaspoon of garlic powder
- One-half of a cup of softened cream cheese
- Salt and fresh cracked black pepper
- Cilantro - add as a garnish on top

Instructions for Baking: Preheat oven to 325 degrees, cook rice according to the details on the package, and once cooked, drain and set aside. Melt butter in a medium-sized pan over medium heat, add the ground meat of your choice and cook for five to seven minutes. Then add the onion and celery and cook for an additional five minutes, and then add salt and pepper to taste. Get a large bowl and add the rice, add the cheese, chiles, sour cream, cream cheese, the meat and veggie mix, and the stock. Also, add the garlic powder and black pepper. Spread the mix out evenly in the baking pan and top off with the leftover cheese. Then proceed to bake at 325 degrees for twenty to twenty-five minutes or until cheese is nice and bubbling. Add the cilantro to garnish and enjoy this simple and delicious meal!

Garlic Butter Chicken Bites with Zucchini Noodles

This is another quick meal to produce that is popular and tasty. It fits in well to most diets even though it is technically a keto meal.

- Three to four boneless and skinless chicken breasts, cut into medium bite-sized chunks

- Four to five medium zucchinis, rinsed and spiralized (or a pack of Zucchini Noodles that you bought at the store)
- Four tablespoons butter, divided up
- Two teaspoons of minced garlic
- One tablespoon of hot sauce - brands may vary
- One-fourth of a cup or sixty milliliters of low sodium chicken broth- bone broth can also be used
- Juice of one half of a lemon
- One tablespoon of minced parsley
- One teaspoon of fresh thyme leaves
- Crushed red chili pepper flakes- option
- Several slices of lemon to use for garnish
- The Marinade
- Two tablespoons of olive oil
- One tablespoon of hot sauce (Sriracha is popular but other brands can be used) or one teaspoon of chili powder
- Two teaspoons of salt
- One teaspoon of fresh cracked black pepper
- Two teaspoons of garlic powder
- One teaspoon of Italian seasoning

Instructions: Cut up the chicken breast into bite-sized pieces and combine with olive oil, pepper, garlic powder, salt, Italian seasoning, chili powder or hot sauce and mix up well in a bowl until it is seasoned evenly, then allow to marinate in the fridge for a half to one hour. Wash zucchini and then use a spiralizer to make the zucchini noodles and then set them aside. Set out the chicken pieces in marinade until they reach room temperature. Stir fry the chicken pieces until they are a golden brown and then remove and set aside. In the same pan over high heat, add two tablespoons of butter, lemon juice, and the hot sauce. Let it simmer and reduce for one to two minutes while stirring regularly. Stir in the minced garlic and fresh parsley and then add in the zucchini noodles. Allow the juices to reduce for a minute if the juice from the zucchini gives out too much water. Finally, add the chicken bites back into the pan and stir for another minute or two to reheat. Add more parsley for garnish along with crushed chili pepper, lemon slices, and fresh thyme. This dish is best if served immediately.

Buttery Garlic Herb Chicken with Lemon Cauliflower Rice

This dish is popular and both keto-friendly and gluten-free. A low-carb dish that is easy and can be made quickly and that the whole family can enjoy.

- One and a half pounds (six hundred and fifty grams) of boneless skinless chicken thighs or breasts
- Two tablespoons of butter
- One teaspoon of chopped fresh thyme and one teaspoon of fresh chopped oregano, one teaspoon of freshly chopped rosemary
- Fourteen ounces of (four hundred grams) of cauliflower rice (one medium head)
- One medium onion, chopped well
- Four garlic cloves, minced well
- One-fourth of a cup (sixty milliliters) of chicken broth
- One tablespoon of hot sauce
- One-half of a cup of grated parmesan cheese
- One-half of a cup fresh chopped parsley
- Juice of one half of a lemon, add zest, and lemon slices for garnishing
- The marinade
- One teaspoon of Italian seasoning
- One tablespoon olive oil
- One teaspoon paprika
- Fresh cracked pepper, to taste
- Juice of one half of a lemon

The Instructions: In a big bowl, set chicken thighs and sprinkle with paprika, Italian seasoning, olive oil, black pepper, and lemon juice. Mix together well and allow to marinate for ten to fifteen minutes. Meanwhile, put the cauliflower florets on pulse in a food processor for about fifteen to thirty seconds or until you obtain a rice-like consistency. Then set this aside for now.

Melt two tablespoons of butter in a medium-sized pan over medium to low heat. Then add the oregano, thyme, and the rosemary. Set the chicken with the skin side down and cook for four to five minutes on each side until the chicken is no longer pink in color and reaches 165°F in temperature. Cooking time will vary a little depending on the size of the chicken thighs. Remove chicken from the pan and set aside. Keep the cooking juices from the chicken thighs and fat in the pan for now. Using the same pan, fry the garlic and the onion for one minute until fragrant but be sure not to burn it. Add in the hot sauce and stir to mix well. Then add the riced cauliflower and mix everything else together. Add in the chicken stock, the parsley, the lemon zest, and lemon juice. Cook for two or three minutes to reduce cooking juices then put in the parmesan cheese. Then proceed to adjust seasoning as it is needed. Put the chicken thighs over cauliflower rice and reheat in a swift fashion. Serve with the fresh, cracked black pepper, red chili pepper flakes, fresh herbs, and more parmesan if you want.

Along with a teaspoon of fresh thyme, be sure it is chopped well.

Super Foods and Intermittent Fasting

Superfoods have certainly been an ongoing rage in the last few years or so, and many of them rightly deserve the title! There are many great foods that go along great with the intermittent fasting lifestyle and several super foods that are particularly useful in aiding with overall health and weight loss. A superfood is considered a food that is very rich in vitamins and minerals and has extra benefits as opposed to a regular food. Some of these superfoods can and will really help you out when you are in your feeding period, as well as overall health and longevity.

Superfood One: Leafy Dark Greens

Dark leafy greens are rich in nutrients, zinc, calcium, iron, and folate just to name a few. What really makes dark leafy greens in the 'super' category is that it has the potential to drastically reduce the risk of certain diseases including type two diabetes and heart disease. Dark leafy greens also contain high levels of anti-inflammatory properties and can actually help to prevent and fight cancer.

Superfood Two: Eggs

Eggs are also a great food that has countless health benefits. High in healthy fat and a great source of protein. They are rich in antioxidants, especially lutein and zeaxanthin. These particular antioxidants collect around the retina of the eye and help protect the eyes from sunlight and macular degeneration. Eggs are also considered one of the most nutrient-rich foods on the planet. They are also rich in phosphorus, selenium, and iron. While they do have cholesterol, it is actually the 'good' cholesterol and helps to lower and consolidate the bad cholesterol in the veins. Interestingly enough, nearly all of the nutrients in eggs are in the yolk. Eggs are a great addition to nearly all diets and go well with the intermittent fasting lifestyle.

Superfood Three: Avocado

Avocados, a beloved, delicious, and incredible superfood. It is a great substitute, great on or with many foods, and a very healthy superfood. It is considered a fruit that is greasy; the grease coming from omega 3 fatty acids which helps break down cholesterol. This is also high in fiber, vitamin D, and folic acid. It has properties to help prevent cataracts and aid with proper digestion. Avocados help to slow down aging and are high in potassium. Basically, there is little not to love about avocados, they are very healthy, go with just about everything and are loaded with good, healthy greases, and antioxidants. The avocado goes great with intermittent fasting. Many people use avocados when breaking a fast or easing back into eating. They have a tough outer skin with a smooth inside and can be spread on food, scooped, and eaten or made into something. Avocados are excellent for health in general.

Superfood Four: Turmeric

Exceptionally popular in the last five or so years. Turmeric has gotten quite the magical reputation. While it is not an end all cure all, it is a superfood with plenty of positive health effects. Turmeric is actually a spice from India that has been used for medicinal purposes of several hundred years. Turmeric has powerful antioxidants and a solid anti-inflammatory property. The downside of turmeric is that it does not absorb into the bloodstream particularly well; however, using black pepper, another spice, does help with that. Since turmeric does not absorb well, it works better against inflammation that is more acute than chronic. Turmeric is a spice and can be used to season or mixed with other foods to get the effects and flavor. Many people that experience daily pain consume turmeric, and it fits in well with many foods and is a great natural supplement. Green tea can help to prevent damage to DNA; it is also able to shut down a specific molecule that has a role in the formation of cancer cells.

Superfood Five: Green tea

Green tea is especially great for the intermittent fasting lifestyle. The tea leaves are steamed which make them high in antioxidants. Green tea can actually help to prevent cancer, in several ways. With females that drink tea, it can help to prevent osteoporosis. Green tea helps to repair damage caused by the liver from alcohol as well. It helps prevent autoimmune disorders, Parkinson's disease, and Alzheimer's. Green tea also has caffeine which is a low-level stimulant and can increase focus. Green tea works very well in an intermittent fasting diet plan because it can be consumed at any time. It does not matter if you are in a fasting period or not. Green tea can be consumed at any point and many women have said how it really helps to get over the hunger periods and ease the transition.

According to studies in Japan, where they are big green tea drinkers, three cups of green tea a day can help to ward off breast cancer and five cups a day and you are up to sixteen percent less likely to develop heart disease. For those dedicated tea drinkers that drink at all hours of the day, decaffeinated version of green tea is also available. Green tea comes in a huge variety of flavors and beneficial to your health no matter if you prefer to drink it hot or cold. For those that are seeking the benefits of green tea but do not like the taste, there are pill forms as well.

Superfood Six: Berries

Berries are a tasty and diverse superfood. Nearly all berries are powerful antioxidants and full of fiber. Usually, the different colors mean they are rich in different vitamins. Blackberries have the highest folate levels with raspberries right behind them. Strawberries are very high in vitamins K and C. Of all the berries, raspberries have the highest fiber count. Nearly all berries are considered superfoods and have good benefits. Berries go great in smoothies, on top of cereal or oatmeal, and can be mixed and blended with many different meals. A great overall healthy food that easily works into a healthy diet.

Conclusion

In conclusion of this guide, we hope that you have learned some of the benefits and have a better understanding of how intermittent fasting, in some form or another, can be beneficial to nearly every woman. The various intermittent fasting methods have been proven to help with many health issues and weight loss, a problem that plagues thousands of women in today's society. There is evidence that is beginning to show that intermittent fasting helps to naturally regulate type two diabetes, heart health, slow down aging and countless other benefits. Every day there is more and more science-backed research showing another benefit, ranging from neurological disease prevention to the evidence that intermittent fasting could potentially help cancer patients.

The beauty of intermittent fasting is that it is more of a lifestyle as opposed to the common diet. Intermittent fasting is much less restrictive as it is focusing on when you eat more than what you eat. You can experiment with what fasting protocol best fits you and your lifestyle. Once you have adjusted to a schedule that works for you, there is nothing left but to enjoy feeling good and having the freedom to do and eat what you like. Intermittent fasting can and has helped a great variety of women to get onto the proper path for leading the healthiest life possible.

Thank you.

www.ingramcontent.com/pod-product-compliance
Lightning Source LLC
Chambersburg PA
CBHW020302030426
42336CB00010B/871